TIBETAN AYURVEDA

In a spirit that honors the great traditions of Tibetan Ayurveda, the book presents the preventive aspects of Tibetan medicine in a form adaptive to the world audience. For readers who sincerely want to assess their lives and make intelligent choices based on Tibetan traditions will find what is offered here easy to follow and beneficial.

TIBETAN AYURVEDA

Health Secrets from the Roof of the World

ROBERT SACHS

New Age Books

ISBN: 978-81-7822-327-8

First Indian Edition: 2009

First published in USA by Healing Arts Press
(A division of Inner Traditions International)
published by arrangement with ITL

Disclaimer:
Note to the reader: This book is intended as an informational guide. The remedies, approaches, and techniques described herein are meant to supplement, and not to be a substitute for, professional medical care or treatment. They should not be used to treat a serious ailment without prior consultation with a qualified health care professional.

Published by
NEW AGE BOOKS
A-44 Naraina Phase-I
New Delhi-110 028 (INDIA)
Email: nab@vsnl.in
Website: www.newagebooksindia.com

For Sale in Indian Subcontinent Only

Printed in India
at Shri Jainendra Press
A-45 Naraina Phase-I, New Delhi-110 028

This book is dedicated to my father, Sherman David Sachs, a veterinarian, who gave me many valuable lessons on preventative health-care. Thanks, Dad.

With much love and appreciation. . .

CONTENTS

ACKNOWLEDGMENTS 11

PREFACE 15

FOREWORD by Dr. Lobsang Rapgay 17

INTRODUCTION 19

I. SELF-EVALUATION 25

- Constitution: Our Blueprint for Well-Being 28
- How to Score the Four Tests 33
- Test 1: Stature and Physical Characteristics 35
- Test 2: General Symptoms 37
- Test 3: Tibetan Personality Profile 41
- Test 4: Specific Symptoms Observed Over Time 47
- Adding Up the Scores 49
- Using the Constitutional Type as a Guide 50

II. NUTRITIONAL PRACTICES 53

- Tastes 55
- Quantities of Food 56
- Seasonal Considerations 57
- Chewing 57
- Food Selection and Preparation 58
- Food Recommendations for the Six Constitutions 60
  - *Nutritional Practices for the LUNG-type Constitution* 60
  - *Nutritional Practices for the TrIPA-type Constitution* 63
  - *Nutritional Practices for the BEKAN-type Constitution* 66
  - *Combination Nyepa Constitutions* 69
- Food Combining 73
- Food Quality and Special Food Groups 75
- Other Environmental Considerations: Water and Air 79

Supplementation: Vitamins, Herbs, and Super Foods 81
Tibetan Urine Testing for Supplements and Medicines 83
Tibetan Precious Pills 85
Digestive Fire 89
Assessing Nutritional Programs 92

III. EXERCISE 93
Exercise for the LUNG Constitution 95
Exercise for the TrIPA Constitution 95
Exercise for the BEKAN Constitution 96
Seasonal Considerations 96
Tibetan Tai Chi and Chi Kung 97
Tibetan Chi Kung 99
Kum Nye 100
Tibetan Rejuvenative Exercises 102
Yantra Yoga 112
Relaxation Therapy 113

IV. SKILLFUL BEHAVIOR 119
General Behavior — Daily Practices 120
Sleep 121
Hygiene 124
Sexual Intercourse and Practices 125
Spiritual Practices — Cultivating True Healthiness 131
Seasonal Behavior 133
Occasional Behavior 137

V. MEDITATION AND SPIRITUAL PRACTICE 141
What Is Meditation? 143
Meditation on Equanimity 144
Healing Meditation -- as taught by Dr. Lobsang Rapgay 147
Individual Spiritual Orientation 153
Dealing with Problems Arising in Meditation 161

VI. DETOXIFICATION AND REJUVENATION 165
Len Nga (Pancha Karma) Therapy) 166
The Techniques 167
Massage and Steam Hydrotherapy 168
The Five Actions 170
Netra Basti 179
Shiro Dhara 183
Tailoring a General Len Nga Therapy Regimen for You 186
Rejuvenation 188
A Len Nga Therapy Case History 190

VII. TIME AND PLACE 195
Setting and Geomancy 196
Timing and Astrology 198
The Elements 203
Ambience and Social Support 212

APPENDIX ONE: Ego and Suffering: A Buddhist View 215

APPENDIX TWO: Theory of the Three Nyepas 223

APPENDIX THREE: A Concise Meditation on Medicine Buddha 227

APPENDIX FOUR: Mewas and Buddhist Spiritual Practice 230

NOTES 232

GLOSSARY 237

BIBLIOGRAPHY 239

RESOURCES 242

INDEX 245

ACKNOWLEDGMENTS

There are many volumes written by authors in both Eastern and the Western traditions that I am indebted to for their diligent work. I have divided the Bibliography so as to credit them in accordance with their specialty.

There are also many teachers I have encountered from various traditions over the years to whom I am indebted. First and foremost are my closest spiritual teachers, the Venerable Khenpo Karthar, Rinpoche, and Chime Rinpoche, who over the years have continued to give me meditation instruction and guidance. Included with Khenpo Rinpoche and Chime Rinpoche is the Venerable Chogyam Trungpa, Rinpoche, whose Shambhala Training has had a profound impact on my meditation practice and the mindfulness in which I engage in all activities of my life. Also, to my dear friend and an excellent lama, Ole Nydahl, who has been able to transform Tibetan Buddhism to fit contemporary Western minds. To these four I am grateful. They provide the source material for much of the spiritual dialogue throughout this book and the overview of meditation practice and its relevance to daily life.

I want to thank my close friend and teacher Rex Lassalle for being an example to me in how to integrate preventive healthcare practices into daily life. His training programs in martial arts exercise and shiatsu prepared me for my training with the late Tibetan tai chi master Liu Siong, whom I also wish to thank. Rex was my benefactor for this training. He also brought me to study macrobiotics with Michio Kushi, whom I consider the buddha of food. It is my macrobiotic training with Michio that has made it possible for me to comprehend and modernize the teachings on nutrition in Tibetan medicine. I also want to thank Michio for introducing me to the teachings on Nine-Star Ki astrology, a system found within Japanese, Chinese, and Tibetan astrology under different names. Material on Nine-Star Ki, called in Tibetan the system of *mewas*, is discussed in the chapter "Meditation and Spiritual Practice" and the final chapter, "Time and Place," on how and when to integrate these practices into daily life. I thank Rex, again, for coaxing me to go deeper into the study of Nine-Star Ki.

From 1981 through 1986, I had the great privilege of working with Dr. Walt Stoll of what was then the Holistic Medical Center in Lexington, Kentucky. A master allopathic physician with a profound respect for natural and holistic therapies, Walt was able to show me how to integrate divergent health practices and philosophies. Stoll is a pioneer and a good friend. I thank him for his example, the patronage that made it possible for me to train in the Medicine Buddha teachings and practice, and his relentless pursuit to find better methods to benefit his patients — even when that means breaking ranks with the convention of the day.

I want to thank the various teachers of Tibetan medicine whom I have encountered: Dr. Yeshe Donden, Venerable Trogawa Rinpoche, osteopath Tom Dummer, and especially Dr. Lobsang Rapgay. It has been under the direct tutelage of Dr. Rapgay that I have not only studied materials from the *Gyud-Zhi* but have come into contact with other works of Tibetan teachers and their students and have been able to integrate other health-related knowledge from years with Khenpo Karthar, Rinpoche, and other masters and to reformulate years of alternative health-care training to fit within the framework of Tibetan medicine. Thus I pay a special tribute to Dr. Rapgay. He is a brilliant teacher and a good friend. Also, many thanks and "*namastes*" to Ayurvedic physicians Vasant Lad, Pakanj Naram, and especially Sunil Joshi. Dr. Joshi has been responsible for deepening my knowledge of the detoxification and rejuvenation practices of Ayurveda common both to Indian and Tibetan Ayurveda and continues to inspire me with his dedication to his clients.

My lifetime companion, Melanie, also deserves a special credit. A pioneer and original thinker, Melanie has often been the captain who has steered our course. Her interest in Ayurveda brought us to a place where we have learned more about the practical side of Tibetan medicine. Her theoretical knowledge is extensive, and her work in the area of beauty and rejuvenation brings Ayurveda to a new level in Western consciousness. In this volume, she has acted as consultant and support. I thank her for her support as a professional and as a wife. I openly proclaim my love and admiration for her as a partner whose hand I am proud to hold on the path of life.

I would also like to thank Thomas Bonner for photography that is the basis for many of the drawings in the book, Pat Hanaway for going through the entire text and offering suggestions for making fundamental concepts in Tibetan medicine clearer to the reader, and my editors, Sara Held and Ann Mason, who have been instrumental in steering this project to completion. Thanks also to Harmon Houghton and Marcia Keegan.

Finally, since I am not a physician, the material I have presented in this book, while it represents years of training, is in no way comparable to the work of someone who has completed the ten to twenty years of study required to become a Tibetan doctor. This book is for preventive health-care purposes only. Although such practices can go a long way toward alleviating the pain and suffering we experience, they are not intended to replace diagnosis and treatment under the care of a competent physician or health-care practitioner of whatever tradition. At the same time, I encourage readers to discuss these practices with their health-care providers when appropriate so that a more extensive, more beneficial knowledge of health care and treatment can emerge for the benefit of all.

PREFACE

My interest in Tibetan medicine began in 1972 when I became involved with Tibetan, or Vajrayana, Buddhism. But it was not until 1977 that my wife Melanie and I were able to pursue this interest when we became part of a Tibetan medical study group in London under the guidance of Dr. Tom Dummer. Other than information on Tibetan medical philosophy and theory, little material about daily health practices in the Tibetan medical system had been translated. However, from my study of other Eastern medical traditions and martial arts, I was convinced that such day-to-day practices must also exist in the Tibetan medical system.

Soon after moving back to the United States from England, I met the Venerable Khenpo Karthar, Rinpoche, abbot of Karma Triyana Dharmachakra in Woodstock, New York. An impeccable teacher with a sixth sense of what needs to be answered beyond the question posed, Khenpo Rinpoche answered all my questions about Oriental medicine, with an explanation of why the question was not a correct one. This process of redefining and refining went on between Khenpo Rinpoche and me for five years. As I look back I see that during that time my understanding of medicine and healing was being steered to a deeper level of awareness with great subtlety.

In 1984, it was announced that Khenpo Rinpoche would be giving a month-long seminar on the practice of the Medicine Buddha. Looking forward to the seminar with great anticipation, I believed that I could finally get all my questions about Tibetan medicine answered.

However, what transpired during the seminar was not at all what I had expected. There were no lectures on anatomy or physiology; nor were there any on food, herbs, medicines, or medicine theory. Instead, our group was given a thorough explanation of the meditation practice on the Medicine Buddha. Day in and day out we learned details of visualization and the importance of the symbology. Day in and day out, we recited hours of Medicine Buddha mantras. Day in and day out, Khenpo Rinpoche reframed our perception of reality, revealing the enlightened nature of all aspects of our existence, taking us beyond what we thought was possible. When it was time to leave, I had learned something far more important than what I had expected, something that was to affect all my future studies of medicine and healing.

In the practice of Medicine Buddha meditation, one visualizes that the teachings of the Medicine Buddha come pouring into one in the form of colors, sounds, and impressions. While engaged in visualization and reciting the mantra, one may consider some health issue for oneself or someone else. Whatever one needs to know flows into one in a similar manner.

When practicing meditation following a spiritual path, there is a point at which one knows that the world is much vaster than normally perceived. Thus a leap of faith is necessary. This leap is supposed to be grounded in confidence, both in the practice and in the teacher empowering one to do the practice. Visualization in the Tibetan Buddhist context is not creative imagery or a mere affirmation of what we want to see. According to tradition, what is visualized is the reality we would know if we were not blinded by our preconceptions.

In this context, from the time I received these teachings from Khenpo Karthar, Rinpoche, and began doing daily recitations of the Medicine Buddha practice, a continuous flow of information regarding both Indian and Tibetan Ayurvedic medicine has been imparted to me in such a manner that I have been able to integrate it into my daily life. The teachers and the published and unpublished materials I have discovered since then have not only deepened my knowledge of Tibetan medicine and healing arts but have also provided me with insights into what I had previously studied about alternative and traditional medical practices.

FOREWORD

Knowledge of the healing science of Tibet is slowly coming to the West as more and more publications in English are being made available to the non-Tibetan reader. Bob Sachs's work *Health for Life* is a major departure from these publications because it not only emphasizes the practical side of Tibetan medicine but also integrates aspects of other related sciences of Tibet, such as Yantra Yoga, meditation, and spiritual practice, in a way that presents a true picture of the holistic nature of Tibetan medicine.

Tibetan medicine was probably the first integrated system of ancient healing sciences. From the seventh through the tenth century, Tibetan kings encouraged physicians from India, China, Nepal, Persia, and Greece to come to Tibet to teach their traditional medical sciences to Tibetan physicians, who were then primarily influenced by shamanic and Ayurvedic systems of medicine. Consequently, in the eleventh century the famous Tibetan physician Yutok Yonten Gonpo produced the four medical tantras, the first major texts on Tibetan medicine, which present Ayurveda, Chinese medicine, and Persian and Greek medicine from a Buddhist philosophical and psychological perspective.

Unfortunately, in the last century Tibetan medicine as science and practice has primarily focused on herbal medicine and limited use of acupuncture while ignoring many other forms of treatment such as *pancha karma*, lifestyle management, and Yantra Yoga. In the last few years I have attempted to revive these aspects of Tibetan medicine in the West, and Bob Sachs has been a very valuable assistant in this process.

For several years Bob Sachs has been studying Tibetan medicine with me and other physicians. Because of this knowledge and his familiarity with other medical science systems, such as Chinese and naturopathic medicine, his book discusses these lesser but equally important parts of Tibetan medicine in a more comprehensive manner than previously. I therefore feel honored to present *Health for Life* and hope that Bob will continue to promote the teachings of the Buddha and the Tibetan healing sciences with the vigor and clarity that reflect the spirit of the Buddhist healer.

As we move into a new age of healing in which reliance on physicians and technology has to be matched by a recognition and trust of our own capacity to heal, we are called upon to acknowledge more and more the relationship between mind, body, and soul as the ultimate basis for genuine healing. This book provides an avenue for incorporating Tibetan healing concepts into our daily lives, not just as an intervention against sickness but as a part of our overall well-being.

Dr. Lobsang Rapgay

INTRODUCTION

The purpose of this book on preventive health care in Tibetan medicine is twofold. First and foremost, in a time when health care has become a major personal, social, and political issue, this book offers useful information for building a balanced lifestyle that promotes health and prevents disease. In the Tibetan medical tradition there is a more comprehensive preventive health-care model than can be found in current Western conventional and alternative health-care models. Diet, exercise, relaxation, environmental consciousness, meditation, rejuvenation, and spiritual growth, all extolled as essential for the promotion of health and personal growth, are part of this great tradition. What makes the Tibetan model even more appealing is that, unlike the current holistic health models, which are a patchwork of insights and practices from various systems, it is an integrated system rooted in one well-formulated philosophical perspective. In the Tibetan system practices done are designed to be complementary, and the logic for various practices within the system is based on a specific philosophy of life and health that extols the importance of balance for creating a healthy, productive, and meaningful life.

The second purpose of this book is linked closely to the first. Until now, proponents of Tibetan medicine have not fully demonstrated how it fits into Western culture and the modern world. Great Tibetan doctors have come to the West. Their interaction with the Western medical community has been written up in medical journals. These doctors have met hundreds, if not thousands, of people as clients, taking pulses and prescribing medicines. Yet while some people have benefited from their guidance, they have not received comprehensive instruction in Tibetan daily health-care and lifestyle practices. This volume is an attempt to change this situation. In a spirit that honors this great tradition, the preventive aspects of

Tibetan medicine are presented in a form adapted to a Western audience. Readers who sincerely want to assess their lives and make intelligent choices based on Tibetan tradition will find what is offered here easy to follow and beneficial.

The primary source for much of the material presented here are the four great medical tantras, called the *Gyud-Zhi.* This is a shortened name for what is translated as "The Ambrosia Heart Tantra: The Secret Oral Teachings on the Eight Branches of the Science of Healing."[1] The word *tantra* literally translated means lineage.[2] It implies a teaching that has been passed on in an unbroken line since the time it was transmitted by an enlightened being to at least the time when the teaching was "officially" put in the written or oral form used since. According to the sacred history of Tibet, tradition teaches that the origin of these tantras is Buddha Vaidurya or Buddha of Aquamarine Light, who first presented them in a paradise known as Tanatuk. In that celestial paradise, Medicine Buddha (as he is commonly known) emanated Himself as two beings: the sage Yile Kye and the sage Rigpe Yeshe. As is customary with many of the Buddha's teachings, the transmission took the form of a dialogue. The sage Yile Kye raised pertinent questions, and the sage Rigpe Yeshe answered them.[3] For those interested in a more secular historical view of events, Terry Clifford's *Tibetan Buddhist Medicine and Psychiatry*[4] provides details on how the *Gyud-Zhi* came from India to Tibet and what influence Tibetan shamanic and medical traditions, as well as knowledge that was passed along the Silk Road, had on the practice and interpretations of the tantras. Of particular note are the medical conferences organized by King Srongtsan Gampo in the eighth century. Physicians were invited from Persia, India, China, and other parts of Asia to share their knowledge of healing, thus enriching Tibetan medical practice and establishing Tibet as the holistic medical capital of Asia.

Whether one prefers the sacred or the secular historical account of the development of Tibetan medicine, the scope and depth of knowledge of anatomy and physiology, diagnosis, and treatment passed on in the *Gyud-Zhi* is extensive and impressive, even by the standards of Western medical science. What is pertinent for the Western reader is to distinguish the four levels of Tibetan medicine that are woven throughout the narrative of these texts.

The first level of medicine has to do with lifestyle changes: diet, exercise, relaxation, and daily, seasonal, and occasional behaviors. It is said that the Tibetan doctor will recommend such changes first unless a more invasive intervention is needed. This principle is very much in keeping with principles of modern holistic medicine; making healthy changes in one's lifestyle goes a long way toward bringing the body back to viable balance, so that it no longer acts as host to whatever illness has beset it. At the same time, because lifestyle change means a change in one's personal habits, with social and psychological repercussions, conventional Western physicians are inclined to approach the subject with trepidation. It means involving the patient in the cure. Inquiring into the patient's lifestyle may be considered an invasion of the patient's privacy. Unfortunately, if such an inquiry is not pursued until after other therapies have been implemented and have failed, the disease may have progressed to the point where lifestyle changes that earlier may have had a great impact and benefit are now either ineffective or meaningless.

Tibetan healers, in contrast, view lifestyle changes as less invasive because they do not involve any radical changes in body chemistry or procedures that would alter the body itself, as is the case with surgery. Thus the Tibetan doctor/healer first offers processes and remedies that will cause the least disruption to the body and energy of a client.

The second level of Tibetan medicine involves the use of herbs and specific medicinal preparations, massage, and techniques that cleanse and rejuvenate the body. In the Orient, Tibet was known as the land of medicinal plants, and Tibetan medicines were highly prized. One of the guiding principles in Tibetan pharmaceutical tradition is that once a proper diagnosis is made, the prescribed medicine (usually an herbal compound) should cause no side effects. Massage and various bodily cleansing practices such as herbal emetics, enemas, and purgatives are done in accordance with body constitution and presenting conditions. Massage is classified as a second-level therapy, more invasive than lifestyle changes, because it involves touching, hence changing the energy of the person being massaged. For Tibetans it is important that the practitioner using massage is medically and ethically competent to effect positive change through touch.

The third level of Tibetan medicine is the most invasive in its physical impact on the body. This includes acupuncture, moxabustion (a form of acupuncture using directed heat rather than needles), bloodletting, and surgery. Tibetans claim to have been the originators of the "golden needle" acupuncture practices but abandoned it as a therapeutic modality, passing it on to the Chinese. Surgery, graphically explained in Tibetan medical texts, was banned when a member of the Tibetan royal family died during an operation. Of the third level, only blood-letting and moxabustion are still actively practiced.

The fourth level of Tibetan medicine is spiritual medicine which utilizes specific rituals performed by the medical practitioner but also involves the patient. One could say that this level permeates all other levels of Tibetan medicine. Clients are asked to reflect on their condition and base their thought and action on religious and ethical principles. The purpose here is to eliminate the negative impressions of the mind and the activities that are often at the root of illness or imbalance.

What we shall be addressing in this volume are primarily the first two levels of Tibetan medicine: that is, lifestyle changes, herbal intervention, cleansing, and rejuvenation as well as the principles of basic meditation and spiritual training that are a part of the fourth level.

In addition to materials gathered from the *Gyud-Zhi* itself, the information in this volume comes from a number of sources, all of which are authentic as far as I can determine. It must be understood that the medicine and healing traditions of Tibet were influenced not only by the introduction of the *Gyud-Zhi*, indigenous Tibetan Bonpo shamanism, and the interfacing with other cultures but also by Tibetan social and cultural heritage, which molded this material in various ways to create local and regional variations in medicine and healing practices.

The great medical college of Chakpori in Lhasa has been the most important source for all of the various aspects that went into creating Tibetan medicine as it is represented to the world. For the most part, however, beyond the cosmopolitan atmosphere of Lhasa, Tibet was comprised of wandering nomadic communities or self-sufficient agrarian villages attached to various monasteries. These monasteries not only gave spiritual inspiration to the people but also trained its monks and lamas to become the doctors and healers for the communities. Because there were few major roads, travel was slow and somewhat hazardous. Thus while basic knowledge, such as that found in the medical tantras, may have remained similar from one locale to the next, local doctors and healers would come to their own unique understanding of that material and, in many cases, innovate in accordance with the needs of the environment and the people they served. Consequently, even today some teachers may not be familiar with Tibetan rejuvenation exercises, tai chi, or *kum nye*, for example or many unique variations or different approaches to the same material or practices.

As Dr. Leon Hammer notes about Chinese medicine in his *Dragon Rises, Red Bird Flies*, in Tibet as in China, it is a misperception to assume that all that is known and practiced was a unified system and known by all "in the field" of medicine and healing.[5] In instances when I have not had direct experience with a certain technique or practice I have reported the benefits that others have experienced through following practices that have been passed on to them as being Tibetan. Tibetans espouse a pragmatic approach to life and experience: Does something work, or doesn't it? In the same spirit, I have included what I consider relevant data from other sources of natural therapies used today. Because of cultural and environmental differences, certain Tibetan healing practices require some adaptation or "updating." Tradition is important insofar as it is relevant to present experience. As times and circumstances change, all traditions must inevitably grow into the present to be useful. My advice to the readers of this book is to take a pragmatic approach. Study, practice, and experience. See how these preventive health-care practices work for you. This is the spirit behind true preventive health care and especially behind Tibetan medicine and its preventive health-care practices.

chapter one

SELF-EVALUATION

The foundation of Tibetan Ayurveda and healing practices is an understanding of our relationship to the world around us. We are not separate from the cosmic and natural forces that exist in all that is created in this universe. The purpose of Tibetan Ayurveda is to gently remind us of this relationship. For when we live and feel at one with the forces within and around us, we have the optimal conditions for healthy life, personal transformation, and the resourcefulness to benefit others.

Tibetan Ayurveda, in keeping with its Buddhist philosophical underpinnings, asserts that we have the innate potential to be like a Buddha. "Buddha" here is meant as a description rather than as a title. We have the potential to be awake and alive in the fullest sense. In truth, our bodies are like rainbows: translucent, yet capable of feats we now only hear of in history, myth, and inspired religious literature. Seen in their fullest splendor, our bodies would not be viewed as mere vessels or containers subject to illness and decay but as physical mechanisms capable of inspiring and touching the lives of others. Our speech and actions have the potential to be spontaneous, direct, and joyful. Our deep yearning for self-fulfillment and the desire to see a better world for ourselves and others is a testimony to the truth of this potential. Through tales or examples in our lives we have known people who have not seemed to be burdened by living and being in the world. Beyond these role models in our lives, we can surely see that when we feel clear and speak and act truthfully, we experience how much energy this gives to us and those around us.

Both our body and our activity potentials are dependent on our minds. In truth, our minds are luminous, clear, and unimpeded in time and space. They are not bound by size, shape, or color. The limitations we impose on our minds, no matter how apparently solid or convincing, are mere fictions that are ephemeral. As we come to know how our minds actually work, we see that all thoughts, all emotions come and go and that the rigid concepts we hold about our physical bodies and the world and objects prevent us from being the luminous light beings that we are. Whatever limits we impose, there is always space around them. This implies that there is always room to grow, to expand, to embrace more and more of our world until we come to the ultimate realization that we are not in the least bit separate from our world. Our minds, bodies, and actions come into total balance and harmony with the world around us. And because our perceptions have been cleared of delusion, we see the world in a new light. Perfection is always there if we were only to wake up to it.

THE THREE POISONS

What prevents us from realizing this perfection is that we fail to see , or we obscure these potentials by abusing them. Misdirected thoughts and actions lead to all the suffering that we experience in our lives. The medical tantras teach that all of our suffering, be it physical, emotional, or spiritual, is caused by what in Buddhism are known as the Three Poisons: attachment, aggression, and ignorance.[1] Not being enlightened, we do not truly know what is going on, we cling to our misperceptions, and tend to be irritated and affronted by those around us who may suggest to us that our version of reality may not be entirely correct. Thus we react in inappropriate ways that further confusion and perpetuate our sense of alienation from ourselves and others. In this alienated state we lose touch with natural laws and begin to choose ungrounded, even chaotic ways of living in the world. This includes even basic survival skills such as knowing how to eat, exercise, relax, behave, communicate, and so forth. We thus reinforce our confusion and its resultant, which inevitably leads to mental and physical illness.

Within each of us there is an essential — although perhaps very dim — knowing that something is not quite right. But being caught up in our attachment to our view, we may deny this instinct within us. The degree of this denial of what we know in our depths to be true is proportional to the amount of suffering and disease we will experience. This may be denial in the present moment, or it can be the residual effect of transgressions born from the Three Poisons experienced in previous existences. We can never fully escape the repercussions of our previous actions. It is usually an awareness of, or disillusion with, our ego-driven version of the world and an initial acceptance of the potentials we may only have vague inklings of that is the first step in our transformation and healing at all levels. Thus the first step of healing is a spiritual one. As part of the healing journey we must take in order to realize our potentials, we need practices to help uproot the Three Poisons.

If we closely examine our lives, it is not hard to see that each one of us possesses the Three Poisons of ignorance, attachment, and aggression. At the same time, because of our experiences and how we have responded to them, one or two of the poisons will tend to be more pronounced in our psychological makeup and way of being. Some of us will be more gripped by attachment, some by aggression, some by ignorance, some perhaps by a combination of ignorance and attachment, some by attachment and aggression, and others by aggression and ignorance. Please bear in mind that each of the poisons, no matter how ingrained, is ephemeral. Each can be transformed. To transform the root cause of all disease is in fact to conquer that which causes suffering. Attachment can be transformed into a mind that is totally compassionate and expresses its quality of being luminous, clear, and unimpeded. Aggression can be transformed into joyous and spontaneous skillful action. Ignorance can be transformed into a panoramic awareness that allows us to experience our rainbow body and the rainbowlike nature of all phenomena. These are some of the potentials hidden behind the Three Poisons.

THE THREE HUMORS (Tibetan: NYEPAS)

Which poison or poisons is dominant will determine not only how we are programmed to perceive our world, but also how we will feel and the expectations we have regarding how our bodies should be and function in the world. Consequently, we shall have tendencies towards certain afflictions more than others. As the Three Poisons become translated into physiological, psychological, and spiritual tendencies they are known as humors, or *nyepas* (pronounced nyay-pah). In Sanskrit these are known as the *doshas*. The names of the three nyepas and their associated poison are:

POISON:	Attachment	Aggression	Ignorance
NYEPA:	LUNG	TrIPA	BEKAN
pronounced	(loong)	(tee-pah)	(bay-gahn)
DOSHA:	Vata	Pitta	Kapha

According to Tibetan Ayurveda, all cosmic and natural forces are classified within the triad of nyepas. Thus the three nyepas are the foundation of our existence, and they are found in each one of us in varying amounts. Variation in their dominance leads to each person having their own unique traits. This affects our stature, build, whether we easily lose or retain weight, the strength of our digestion, the shape of our eyes, hands, and other features, which organs are strong and which will be weak or problematic, emotions, what illusions are likely to arise when we are unbalanced, and which of the poisons will need to be primarily addressed in our mental development and daily physical care to promote wellness and spiritual development.[2]

CONSTITUTION (Tibetan: Rang-Zhin)
Our Blueprint for Well-Being

Our unique mix of the nyepas forms our basic constitution, what in Tibetan is known as *rang-zhin*. The rang-zhin is like this lifetime's blueprint. If we come to know which of the poisons is dominant in our constitution, we have a reference point from which to build a sane, healthy lifestyle that will support our efforts in efficiently and effectively aiming our life force towards true happiness and enlightenment. A more theoretical description of the theory of the three nyepas and an explanation of how mind states and the Three Poisons affect our psycho-physical makeup are found in Appendix One and Appendix Two.

In Tibetan Ayurveda, there are seven basic constitutional types. Three are one-nyepa dominant constitutions, three are two-nyepa dominant constitutions, and one constitution has all three nyepas in perfect balance. This latter constitution type implies that all poisons have been transformed. This is the manifestation of a saint or bodhisattva.

As the greater portion of this chapter is devoted to the reader finding out what their own constitution is, the following general descriptions of the three one-nyepa constitutions are offered. The purpose here is to help the reader get a sense of how to look at their traits in a collective, holistic manner.

LUNG-type dominant constitution arises from a predominance of attachment to this world. Such a person has a quick, bright mind, which, if imbalanced, becomes flighty, perhaps spaced out, or obsessional. They can be indecisive and worried. Physically, they are akin to the ectomorph in Western physiology. They can be tall and skinny. Or they can be very short. Even if they are of a normal stature, they will have anomalous features; perhaps they will have hands, feet, jaw, torso, or eyes that seem disproportionate to the rest of their body. They thrive in warm, moist, peaceful environments and do worse in environments that are cold, dry, and chaotic. They can be most disturbed by the wind. Their hair is usually dark, perhaps brittle, but of a usual thickness, and they can have the greatest problems of all the constitutions with dryness of the skin. Typical health symptoms they exhibit are bloating, gas, constipation, pains that move from one part of the body to another, and a tendency towards difficulties and pains in their joints. They have the greatest tendency of all the constitutions to experience mental imbalances. They can be energy junkies who want but are disturbed by having constant change and stimulating events. Their energy level is variable. They can go along fine, wake up the next day feeling like they can't even get out of bed, then fine again the next day as if for no apparent reason.

When balanced, the LUNG-type constitution person is brilliant, compassionate, and inspiring to be around.

TrIPA-type dominant constitution arises from a predominance of aggression. Such a person is a critical thinker and decisive. They want to know what is going on but can go to an excess in being "control freaks." They are often identified as the Type A personality. These are the athletic types, most associated with the mesomorph of Western physiology. Well proportioned, they often have fair skin, light-colored eyes, and hair that is blond, red, prematurely grey or white, or thinning. They freckle in the sun and may have a noticeable sensitivity to bright light. They do better in temperate, cooler climates as they are hot blooded. They do worse in very hot humid weather but often love to sweat in the intensity of the heat. These are people who usually tend to push things to an extreme — "to the max." They want to do things when they want to do them; thus they can be pushy and rebellious to a beneficial routine. They often like foods that are the worst for them, like chili, coffee, alcohol, meat, and spicy things. The TrIPA-type can withstand a great deal of physical stress, but if they crack, the physical damage may be extensive as a result of not paying attention to or denying early warning signs. Such signs can be migraines, a tendency towards diarrhea, reproductive tract problems, and various inflammation-type conditions.

When balanced, the TrIPA-type is joyful, dynamic, and magnetizing to those around them.

BEKAN-type dominant constitution arises from a predominance of ignorance about this world. Such a person is slow, methodical, and thorough. If imbalanced, they can become lackadaisical and inert. If pushed too far (which takes a lot as they are very tolerant people), because their mind energy is strong they can be the type that is very resentful and holds deep grudges. Physically, they are associated with the endomorphs — rounded, stocky types with dense bones, thick tissues, large eyes, and way of moving that gives you the impression that all their joints are well lubricated. They almost glide through space. Thus of all the constitutions they can endure the most physically and by and large feel no sense of physical threat from those around them. At the same time, they have a tendency towards laziness, which means they will get less stimulation or physical activity than they really need. They may have a sweet tooth, and certainly have a tendency to put on weight more easily than other constitutions. They can just look at food and put on weight. Such people can have problems that are the result of overburdening their stomach and thus blocking their lymphatic systems. Excess mucus and catarrh are classic BEKAN symptoms. These people do well in environments that stimulate them to move.

When balanced, the BEKAN-type person is generous, kind, tolerant, and projects a sense of security

Of course, such descriptions are overly simplistic, but will hopefully be a starting point for all who wish to explore their nyepa dominance more thoroughly through the tests provided in this chapter.

In Tibetan medicine, knowing a person's constitution, or rang-zhin, is essential to find an effective cure for any symptoms that may arise. Its holistic approach offers different levels of healing intervention depending on how acute or chronic symptoms are. The role of a Tibetan doctor is to restore one's rang-zhin when one experiences imbalance and disease and to maintain that person in balance with his or her rang-zhin. The closer we are able to stay to our original blueprint, the more quickly we will come to know ourselves, what we need to work on, and what means are most effective for us. Thus our path for transformation from our self-limiting reality to the awakening of our potentials is more straightforward and our efforts more streamlined. It is for this reason that physicians of Tibet were not only medically trained in the sense that we use in the West but spiritually trained as well. The doctor must have the outlook of a bodhisattva, a saint, seeing as his or her aim the alleviation of suffering and the promotion of health and healthy conditions so that the patient attains the optimal healthy state: enlightenment.

DISCOVERING YOUR RANG-ZHIN

A truly accurate determination of constitution is a fine art in Tibetan medicine and involves a good deal of preparation on the part of the patient and skill on the part of the physician.[3] In a self-help book such as this, it is not possible to expect the reader to determine their constitution with such depth and accuracy. Still, the result one gets from the tests will give an adequate estimation to set out in the right direction when choosing the right diet, exercise, and lifestyle practices and regimens recommended in this book.

This information should not be used for treating medical conditions. These should be referred to a competent Tibetan Ayurvedic or Indian Ayurvedic health practitioner and your current health support network. However, it is my observation that by merely making changes in accordance with one's rang-zhin, one's own strengths and weaknesses, many of the acute and chronic symptoms of physiological and psychological dis-ease can be alleviated. It can also remove us from a state of dependency on others for our well-being to a state of self-empowerment, in which we learn to become more biologically, psychologically, and spiritually responsible for our lives and the direction our lives take. In this spirit, physicians and competent health practitioners and spiritual teachers become allies in attaining well-being.

It is helpful to approach the following constitutional questionnaires when you are feeling relatively well. You should be in a relaxed and self-reflective (but not morose) state of mind. For a few days try to keep your daily routines as uneventful as possible: typical rising and sleeping times, the usual work load, the usual daily activity. As we Westerners tend to see food as entertainment, this is one area in which we may need to be a little more strict: avoid foods that are very hot or spicy; avoid exceedingly hot or cold drinks; abstain from alcohol and drugs. If you take caffeinated beverages, keep them to a standard level to avoid withdrawal symptoms. After three days of these lifestyle and dietary precautions, approach the self-diagnosis material.

There are four sections of questions broken down into individually scored tests. Some of the questions you answer here will not vary over time; some might. Questions on the Stature and Physical Characteristics Test will remain constant, while physical symptoms and psychological attitudes may change. The

Physical Symptoms Test should be looked at from the standpoint of what you are experiencing now and what you observe to be your overall symptoms during the course of your life. The psychological questions in the Tibetan Personality Profile Test may need to be answered in the present, three months from now, and then after another three months. The reason for this is that our psychological attitudes and opinions about ourselves can change depending on physical health and lifestyle/stress factors. Taking the Tibetan Personality Profile Test three times will give a much truer score. This does not mean that when you add up the scores in the various tests, the Tibetan Personality Profile Test will dramatically skew the results. The changes over the nine-month period are not that extreme, and totaling the scores is designed to take variation into account, as some tests are counted more heavily. Thus your first score on the diagnostic tests will give you a sufficiently accurate reading of your constitution so that you can make changes. After practicing these new behaviors for nine months, when you come to retest you will find that your answers refine your scores and lead you closer and closer to your exact constitutional type.

HOW TO SCORE THE FOUR TESTS

1. For Test 1, Stature and Physical Characteristics, and Test 2, General Symptoms, place a check before the characteristic or symptom you identify with in whatever column it appears. Then tally the checks in the columns. The respective tests ask for your *raw* totals.

2. For Test 3, Tibetan Personality Profile, and Test 4, Specific Symptoms, your answers are graduated. Mark the respective characteristic or symptom in the following manner:

TIBETAN PERSONALITY PROFILE	SPECIFIC SYMPTOMS
3 = characteristic you most identify with	3 = ongoing or frequent complaint
2 = characteristic you sometimes exhibit	2 = sometimes a complaint
1 = characteristic you seldom exhibit	1 = infrequent or not a complaint

Tally the columns at the end of each test and enter your *raw* totals.

3. Mathematically convert each test so that the score of each column is a percentage of 100. For example, let's say that at the end of Test 3 the numbers in the columns are: (raw total)

$$95 \qquad 75 \qquad 45$$

Add these three numbers to get a sum total of points or common denominator:

$$95 + 75 + 45 = 215$$

Now multiply each of the raw totals by 100 and divide each one individually by the sum total or denominator number:

$$\frac{9500}{215} \qquad \frac{7500}{215} \qquad \frac{4500}{215}$$

Place these percentage numbers under the raw scores where you are asked for *percentage* totals.

4. The exceptions in these calculations will be Test 1 and Test 4. After figuring out the percentage numbers for each column in Test 1, double them and enter that number in the percentage total section for Test 1. This test is the most important for determining your rang-zhin. For Test 4, multiply each one of the column numbers that you have converted into a percentage by 0.75. This test counts for three-fourths of a test. The reason for this is given later.
5. Take the numbers you have entered in the section of each test called "percentage totals" (adjusting Test 1 and Test 4) and enter them at the end of the four tests where it says "Adding Up the Scores." To find your particular constitutional mix, follow the remainder of the instructions provided at the end of the tests.

TEST 1: STATURE AND PHYSICAL CHARACTERISTICS

Place a check mark next to the descriptions that fit you best.

	COLUMN 1 (LUNG)	COLUMN 2 (TrIPA)	COLUMN 3 (BEKAN)
FRAME	( ) thin-boned (ectomorphic)	( ) moderate-boned (mesomorphic)	( ) dense-boned (endomorphic)
FEATURES	( ) irregular (i.e., large or small hands, feet, face, jaw, eyes)	( ) proportional (classically athletic)	( ) rounded
WEIGHT	( ) variable (low or watery type overweight appearance)	( ) moderate	( ) overweight (or tendency toward)
EYES:			
Size	( ) small (or uncharacteristically large)	( ) moderate	( ) large (but proportional)
Quality	( ) shifting, dull (drooping eyelids)	( ) sharp, lustrous	( ) beautiful and moist
Lashes	( ) scanty, dry	( ) scanty, but oily	( ) thick, oily
Iris	( ) dark, gray-brown or black	( ) light eyes (blue or green) with yellowish red present	( ) pale, blue or black
Whites	( ) reddish, muddy (red lines in whites)	( ) reddish (more pronounced, also lines)	( ) very white
Other	( ) high eyebrows	( ) sensitive to light	( ) eyes bulge
SKIN:			
Texture	( ) rough	( ) soft	( ) thick
Moisture	( ) dry	( ) slightly oily	( ) oily
Temperature	( ) cool	( ) warm	( ) cool/clammy
Color	( ) variable, brown, black	( ) fair (pink, yellowish, freckles, most sensitive to sun)[1]	( ) pale, whitish
MOUTH:			
Lips	( ) thin (bottom lip may be bigger)	( ) balanced (moderate thickness)	( ) thick
Teeth	( ) protruding, variable in size (big or small for mouth), crooked	( ) moderate size	( ) strong, very white

TEST 1: STATURE AND PHYSICAL CHARACTERISTICS *(continued)*

Jaw	( ) excess tension or looseness in jaw	( ) strong, distinctive	( ) strong
Tongue			
Color	( ) reddish	( ) yellowish	( ) pale, almost colorless
Texture	( ) coarse	( ) slightly slippery	( ) thick, sticky
Coating	( ) minimal	( ) slightly furry	( ) very furry
General Symptoms	( ) pips along rim, lines and cracks on tongue	( ) yellow under tongue where should be blue	( ) generally thick and sticky
Other	( ) trembling, may need to swallow a lot to keep tongue moist	( ) in morning, tongue makes mouth taste bitter on swallowing	( ) thick coating in morning
HAIR:			
Color	( ) dark brown, black	( ) blond, red, premature grey or white	( ) dark or light shades
Moisture			
Oiliness	( ) dry	( ) moderately oily	( ) very oily
Texture	( ) brittle, kinky	( ) soft, straight	( ) wavy
Quantity	( ) normal, moderate	( ) thinning, tendency toward baldness	( ) thick
RAW TOTALS	____________	____________	____________
PERCENTAGE *(Note: double these scores)*			
TOTALS	____________	____________	____________

TEST 2: GENERAL SYMPTOMS

The first symptoms to be discussed require careful observation over time. If you have never paid attention to such symptoms, do so over the next few days while maintaining the regimen suggested above.

THE PULSE: Pulse taking is an art that takes the Tibetan doctor years to master. At our wrists there are pulse tones that can determine the health of each of our organs, our overall constitution, our present condition, and our future. The pulse is even used for purposes of divination. Pulses are classified in accordance with the level of information that is being sought by the pulse taker: constitutional pulses, seasonal pulses, and divinatory pulses, the latter being the way in which the tone, rate, and quality of the pulses can be used to determine life span, specific ailments brought on by various causes (diet, environment, spirits), even the time of death.

Dr. Yeshe Donden gives a concise description of how to take the pulse (this method can be done by oneself, although it is useful to have a friend confirm your results):

> The best place for reading the pulse is about half an inch from the crease at the wrist, on the radial artery [on the thumb side of the wrist, on the front rather than the back of the forearm]. The index, middle, and ring fingers [if doing yourself, of the opposite hand] are to be placed [gently] in a straight line on the radial artery, half an inch from the crease of the wrist. They should not touch each other but should also not be far apart — the distance between them being that of the width of a grain [i.e., rice or barley].[4]

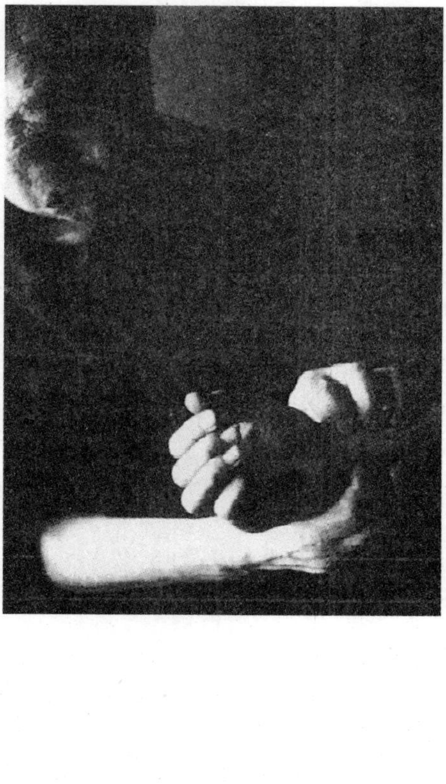

Choje Lama, Tibetan doctor, taking pulses.

Although when doing a complete pulse diagnosis gentle but varying pressure is used, for this test, allow all three fingers to press gently down on the radial artery. Allow about fifteen seconds for your pulse to adjust to the pressure. Then observe the quality of the pulse. Bear in mind that your efforts will yield approximate results. As accurate constitutional pulses are measured when a person is generally in good health, please bear in mind that for your measurement to be useful you should be in relatively good health when you take your pulse. In *Health Through Balance*, Dr. Donden gives an excellent description of the significance of the constitutional pulse beyond classifying it in accordance with the three nyepas.[5]

Be sure to take the pulse in this manner at both wrists.

If taking the pulse is something that you do not feel you can do accurately enough, ignore this particular part of the test and complete the rest of it.

	(LUNG)	(TrIPA)	(BEKAN)
PULSE TYPE	( ) thick, bulky, noticeable at skin level. When you press on it a bit more firmly, the pulse collapses (stops), then continues on as before when you take the pressure off. The number of beats is variable, but more to the slow side — 5 to 6 beats per cycle of respiration. Has a swinging quality.	( ) thin, quick, and tight. More like 7 beats to each respiration cycle. When you press on it, it resists pressure, continuing to beat.	( ) slow, weakly felt. You have to press deep to feel it. Below 4 beats for each cycle of respiration.

Sometimes your pulse will not fit the descriptions as given. In fact, because many people are dominant in more than just one nyepa, there is a good likelihood that the pulse will fit one of the following descriptions more.

	(LUNG/BEKAN)	(LUNG/TrIPA)	(BEKAN/TrIPA)
MIXED PULSE. . .	( ) is deep, long and slow, but stops on pressure (indicate checks for columns 1 and 3 when calculating)	( ) is superficial, fast and thin but stops on pressure (indicate checks for columns 1 and 2 when calculating)	( ) is slow, deep, and a little thick, becoming tighter and resistant to added pressure (indicate checks for columns 2 and 3 when calculating)

URINE: The urine examined here is the midstream of the first morning urination. Although it can be examined by observation in the commode, it is best to pass this sample into a clear jar for more accurate observation.

	(LUNG)	**(TrIPA)**	**(BEKAN)**
Viscosity	( ) watery	( ) oily, possible scum on surface	( ) milky, slightly thick
Temperature	( ) moderate steam	( ) steamy (hottest)	( ) minimal steam
Odor	( ) slight	( ) pungent	( ) none
Color	( ) bluish white hue	( ) reddish or deep yellow	( ) colorless
Bubbles ***(shake sample)***	( ) big bubbles, that dissolve while small ones remain	( ) small, profuse bubbles that disappear almost instantly	( ) profuse small bubbles that stick together and to side of jar and last a long time

SYMPTOMS:

PHYSIOLOGICAL PROCESSES WHERE GENERAL WEAKNESSES ARE OBSERVED:

(LUNG)	**(TrIPA)**	**(BEKAN)**
( ) neurological	( ) endocrine	( ) digestive
( ) psychological	( ) vascular	( ) fluids of the body (i.e. urine, semen, chyle, feces, marrow)

ORGANS AND AREAS WHERE SYMPTOMS TEND TO ARISE:

Try to look back over the course of your life to date and, as accurately as possible, account for all symptoms which tend to show a prevalence or noticeable pattern in your life.

(LUNG)	**(TrIPA)**	**(BEKAN)**
( ) nervous system	( ) small intestine	( ) stomach
( ) heart	( ) liver	( ) spleen/pancreas
( ) lungs	( ) gallbladder	( ) kidneys
( ) colon	( ) veins, arteries, and capillaries	( ) bladder
( ) skin	( ) endocrine glands and reproductive organs	( ) lungs
( ) joints	( ) secretory organs (sweat glands, tear ducts)	( ) lymph and lymph nodes

The general symptoms you experience may cross over all three columns. You are encouraged to check all symptoms and organs where you have experienced stress and/or disease. There are three reasons for this. First, Westerners tend to have mixed-nyepa constitutions. Spiritually, it could be said that Westerners need to address a broader spectrum of mind poisons. From a more mundane perspective, many ethnic and racial lines have been blurred. Thus the dominance of the nyepas of a particular race or culture is altered. Second, our mobility has led us to eat differently and to live in environments different from our ancestors. Moreover, Westerners have experienced more radical medical interventions than were known or experienced by Tibetans. Thus our overall health and function may have been compromised sufficiently to alter our constitutional potentials. Thus this test is not doubled.

	(LUNG)	(TrIPA)	(BEKAN)
RAW TOTALS	________	________	________
PERCENTAGE TOTALS	________	________	________

TEST 3: TIBETAN PERSONALITY PROFILE

The following test was originally presented in its English form by Dr. Lobsang Rapgay. I have modified the language to make it more usable in a Western context. Some questions repeat earlier ones. However, for the purpose of maintaining the integrity of the test, they are included and should be answered.

A numerical value should be given for your answers: **3 = most like you, 2 = sometimes like you, and 1 = rarely like you.** In this test, *leave no spaces in any columns blank.*

It has been my observation from administering this test to individuals and classes that it is the most difficult to be objective about, simply because we spend much of our psychological time projecting and/or being unaware of how we relate to our world. It is for this reason that I encourage people to be reflective and honest and to perform the test at least three times for the best result. When done in this spirit, the Tibetan Personality Profile Test is an accurate and excellent tool.

Remember: 3 = most like you, 2 = sometimes like you, and 1 = rarely like you.

	(LUNG)	**(TrIPA)**	**(BEKAN)**
I. Which of the following traits are basically true of your personality?			
	( ) emotionally respond to situations	( ) rationally respond to situations	( ) deeply consider response to situations
	( ) possessive/clinging	( ) proud/pushy	( ) humble
	( ) variable/generally preoccupied	( ) self-serving	( ) self-denying/ altruistic
	( ) find it difficult to be straightforward	( ) demanding/confrontational	( ) open and avoid hurting others
	( ) unpredictable	( ) predictable	( ) calm and passive
	( ) creative	( ) goal oriented	( ) content with how things are
	( ) many ideas	( ) few but good, practical ideas	( ) not many ideas
SECTION TOTALS	________	________	________
II. How do you relate to people?			
	( ) feel comfortable only under favorable circumstances	( ) seek the company of like-minded people	( ) feel most comfortable when making others happy
	( ) dependent on others	( ) self-reliant (depend on yourself)	( ) OK whether alone or with others

Test 3: Tibetan Personality Profile *(continued)*

	( ) inconsistent, thus unreliable	( ) can be relied on best when your interests are being served	( ) can always be relied on
	( ) argumentative	( ) critical of others	( ) understanding
SECTION TOTALS	________	________	________

III. What is your attitude towards material possessions?

	( ) ambivalent; generally possessive (comfort oriented)	( ) seek material luxuries and wealth (power oriented)	( ) though do not seek material wealth acquire easily (generally content)
SECTION TOTALS	________	________	________

IV. What is your attitude toward spirituality?

	( ) very important	( ) not absolutely necessary	( ) important
	( ) practice intensely on and off	( ) do not find a a need (other priorities)	( ) practice, but not regularly
	( ) changeable faith	( ) if practice, strong faith (zealous)	( ) steady faith
SECTION TOTALS	________	________	________

V. When solving problems, do you tend to

	( ) seek advice from various people and rely on those who seem most comforting	( ) seek advice only from those whom you admire	( ) not seek advice
	( ) be pessimistic and worried	( ) want to settle the problem at once (i.e., right now)	( ) be optimistic regardless of whether you work on the problem or not
	( ) preoccupy yourself with many thoughts and activities (i.e., busy yourself)	( ) work at the problem until solved	( ) delay in working on the problem in the hope that it will solve itself

	( ) brood extensively over a problem	( ) look at things pragmatically	( ) not worry about the problem at all
SECTION TOTALS	________	________	________

VI. How do you relate to new situations and people?

	( ) always involved in many situations with many preconceptions	( ) very selective, with clear preconceptions	( ) rarely involved with either
	( ) anxious and anticipating	( ) look forward to in an aggressive way (wants things to happen now)	( ) slow and steady (things will just happen when they do)
SECTION TOTALS	________	________	________

VII. What are your attitudes about situations in your life that provide you with meaning/ purpose?

	( ) frequent questioning and doubts	( ) pride and satisfaction	( ) contentment with how things are
	( ) impulsive	( ) always looking for new opportunities	( ) avoid new challenges
SECTION TOTALS	________	________	________

VIII. When under stress, what are your general responses?

	( ) anxiety and worry	( ) aggression	( ) lethargy
	( ) insecurity	( ) anger	( ) denial (ignore the situation)
	( ) worry	( ) irritability	( ) procrastination
	( ) mood swings	( ) jealousy (righteous indignation)	( ) letting things be the way they are
	( ) muscular tension	( ) headaches	( ) dullness and heaviness
	( ) hyperventilation	( ) nausea	( ) body feels cold
	( ) frequent sighing	( ) heartburn and acidity	( ) feel like nothing is being digested
SECTION TOTALS	________	________	________

TEST 3: TIBETAN PERSONALITY PROFILE *(continued)*

IX. What level of exercise/exertion do you prefer?

	( ) variable, depending on mood	( ) strenuous, even to point of exhaustion	( ) minimal
	( ) light exercise	( ) competitive exercise and sports	( ) minimal exertion
SECTION TOTALS	______	______	______

X. How is your sleep pattern?

	( ) easily disturbed	( ) need very little	( ) heavy and prolonged
SECTION TOTALS	______	______	______

XI. What is your experience of hunger?

	( ) hunger pangs that come on quickly	( ) hearty appetite without hunger pangs, but do not like waiting when ready to eat	( ) tend to eat, even without much appetite
SECTION TOTALS	______	______	______

XII. What is your normal intake of food?

	( ) variable	( ) regular, regemented	( ) frequent small meals (love to snack)
SECTION TOTALS	______	______	______

XIII. What types of food do you like?

	( ) sweet and sour taste; cabbages, cauliflower, milk, cookies, wheat, yogurt	( ) salty, sweet, and hot tastes; broccoli brown rice, eggs, beans, peaches	( ) hot, sour, and bitter; garlic, ginger, vinegar, miso
SECTION TOTALS	______	______	______

XIV. How long after a meal do you feel some discomfort?

	( ) 2 to 4 hours later	( ) ½ to 2 hours later	( ) immediately after
SECTION TOTALS	______	______	______

XV. Do you experience discomfort in the following environments?

	( ) high altitude and windy	( ) low altitude, hot and dry	( ) wet and humid
SECTION TOTALS	________	________	________

XVI. Which region of your body is the weakest and most susceptible to discomfort and complaints?

	( ) below the navel and to the feet	( ) between the navel and heart	( ) above the level of the heart
SECTION TOTALS	________	________	________

XVII. How do you tend to speak normally?

	( ) rapid, shrill, somewhat rambling	( ) clear, precise, somewhat too sharply to the point	( ) slow and monotonous
SECTION TOTALS	________	________	________

XVIII. Does your body frame tend to be

	( ) thin and bent	( ) medium and muscular	( ) large and heavyset
SECTION TOTALS	________	________	________

TEST 3: TIBETAN PERSONALITY PROFILE —TOTALS FOR ALL SECTIONS *(continued)*

TOTALS FOR ALL SECTIONS:

	LUNG	TrIPA	BEKAN
I.			
II.			
III.			
IV.			
V.			
VI.			
VII.			
VIII.			
IX.			
X.			
XI.			
XII.			
XIII.			
XIV.			
XV.			
XVI.			
XVII.			
XVIII.			
RAW TOTALS			
PERCENTAGE TOTALS			

TEST 4: SPECIFIC SYMPTOMS OBSERVED OVER TIME

In a time when cultures and nations were homogeneous and diet and lifestyle patterns were more in keeping with one's immediate environment, the symptoms one experienced were likely to be aberrations, whether as a result of unusual events, psychological and spiritual disturbances, or lifestyle indulgences or deficiencies. Thus specific symptoms were more than likely to be in keeping with or not far from what one would expect considering one's constitution.

Today, conditions are far more erratic. Cultures and nations intermingle. More people travel. Diet and lifestyle patterns in the West are based more on preference than necessity or logic. Our use of energy, electric and nuclear, has created endless variations of electromagnetic and radioactive stimuli that we are constantly being exposed to. Our exposure to toxic waste and chemicals in the air and drinking water compounds all these factors. In sum, our environment is more stressful than ever before in human history.

According to predictions made by the fourth historical Buddha, Sakyamuni, we are in a period when illnesses experienced are due to an imbalance of the LUNG nyepa. In a time of vast and rapid change on a global level, we need to be able to adapt rather than be attached to habitual ways of thinking and being. As mentioned earlier, LUNG is associated with the poison of attachment. The presence of LUNG symptoms tend to overshadow even our constitutional tendencies. It makes complete sense, therefore, that in both Indian and Tibetan Ayurveda, it is said that the first thing that needs to be addressed when helping oneself or others to relieve distress and promote health is the balancing of LUNG.

Although we are most aware of symptoms, they are in fact the least reliable indicators of our constitution. Thus when the scores of this test are compiled, only three-fourths of the total will be used in our final calculations.

In this test, we are interested not only in a specific symptom but also in how frequently you experience the symptom. Thus, we ask that you ascribe a number value to each symptom. **3 = Frequently; 2 = Sometimes; 1 = Rarely.** If you never experience the symptom, leave the space blank.

TEST 4: SPECIFIC SYMPTOMS OBSERVED OVER TIME

	(LUNG)	(TrIPA)	(BEKAN)
	( ) tremors	( ) dry mouth	( ) cold hands/feet
	( ) lightheadedness and dizziness	( ) bad breath (bitter taste)	( ) heavy/weak hands or feet
	( ) blurred vision, ringing in ears, or olfactory sensitivity	( ) eyes become red or yellowish (jaundice)	( ) indigestion ( ) excess mucus ( ) lethargy
	( ) overtalkativeness	( ) discomfort/pain in liver/gallbladder region	
	( ) diffused (traveling, pain	( ) back pain (localized)	( ) low-grade pain, more gradual and constant
	( ) chills	( ) intense, specific pain, gets worse rapidly	
	( ) tension headaches	( ) migraines	( ) congestive-type headaches
	( ) gas and bloating	( ) nausea	( ) constant full feeling
	( ) constipation	( ) diarrhea	( ) vomiting
	( ) anxiety, delirium	( ) strong smell in urine	( ) frequent belching
	( ) forgetfulness, spaciness		( ) face pale and/or puffy
	( ) insomnia		
	( ) face is dry	( ) face is greasy	
	( ) dry, red skin	( ) oily skin	( ) clammy skin
	( ) dry tongue	( ) feeling of being overheated	( ) loss of appetite
	( ) heart palpitations	( ) strong body odor	( ) loss of sense of taste
Pain or Symptoms Worse:	( ) when hungry	( ) while eating	( ) after eating
Environmental and Lifestyle Factors Present:	( ) eat light, raw, and coarse foods	( ) eat hot, spicy, and stimulants (caffeine, alcohol)	( ) eat heavy, greasy foods
	( ) much emotional upset, especially grief	( ) violent behavior or aggressive atmosphere	( ) damp, cold environment (especially where sleepin)

THE AGE FACTOR — In looking at specific symptoms, age must be considered, especially if you notice that over time certain symptoms have become more noticeable. No matter what our rang-zhin, from infancy through puberty, BEKAN is more accentuated in the constitution and resulting conditions; from puberty to approximately age 55, TrIPA; and from age 55 onward, LUNG. To mitigate age as a factor, subtract 3 points from the BEKAN column if you are at or below puberty, 3 points from TrIPA if you are age 13 to 55, and 3 points from the LUNG column if you are over age 55.

RAW TOTALS			
PERCENTAGE TOTALS			

(Multiply the percentage numbers by 0.75 and enter below)

ADDING UP THE SCORES: Take each of the Percentage Totals from each test and place in the appropriate columns below.

Stature Test			
Personality Test			
General Symptoms			
Specific Symptoms			
TOTALS			

Divide each of the column totals by 4.75.

TOTALS	**(LUNG)**	**(TrIPA)**	**(BEKAN)**
(after division)			

These final figures are the percentages that relate to your constitutional mix — that is, how much LUNG, TrIPA, and BEKAN you are.

For more information, consult Dr. Robert Svaboda's *Prakruti* (see Bibliography). His descriptions of the constitutional types are entertaining and informative.

USING THE CONSTITUTIONAL TYPE AS A GUIDE

Previously mentioned , if you live in accordance with your constitution, life will be more workable. Eating, sleeping, and behaving in accordance with what nurtures you and promotes healthy functioning will allow you to be more focused, relaxed, and successful. In understanding your mix of the Three Poisons, attachment (LUNG), aggression (TrIPA), and ignorance (BEKAN), you will know yourself better and thus be able to study, contemplate, and practice psychological and spiritual techniques to create a more awakened state of being.

When the percentages of one of the test columns is very pronounced, this indicates a one-nyepa constitution: LUNG, TrIPA, or BEKAN, with the other nyepas being less significant with regard to overall health. When the percentages in two of the total columns are very similar, this means that you are a two-nyepa constitution: LUNG-TrIPA, TrIPA-BEKAN, or LUNG-BEKAN. The percentages might be reversed just enough to make some slight variation (TrIPA-LUNG, BEKAN-TrIPA, or BEKAN-LUNG). The seventh type is the one in which all three nyepas are in balance: LUNG-TrIPA-BEKAN.

Of the first six mentioned, it is the interaction between the less dominant and the more dominant, or the competition between two dominant nyepas, that accounts for variations in symptoms and resultant suggested therapies. For those of you dominated primarily by one nyepa, following the recommendations for that nyepa will be most beneficial. For those of you who have two nyepas that dominate, there are combination recommendations that work. Because of specific time and circumstances, symptoms of one nyepa of the two may become more dominant. The way to address that dominance is to follow the recommendations that ameliorate symptoms for that nyepa and then resume the general recommendations. (A simple example: if you are LUNG-TrIPA and you are getting TrIPA symptoms, follow recommendations that help TrIPA conditions until balance is restored.)

The last constitution mentioned — where LUNG, TrIPA, and BEKAN dominate equally — is rare. As stated earlier, this is the constitution of a bodhisattva, or saint. It is said that such a being has conquered the Three Poisons of ignorance, attachment, and aggression. As such, in their awakened state, they use the elements as they see fit in order to help others out of their suffering.

Tibetan Ayurveda asserts that if we practice health and healing methods that are tailored to our rang-zhin, we are certain to get the best results. Dr. Vasant Lad, one of the foremost proponents of Ayurveda in America, in his presentations on Ayurveda, would always ask the question, "But for whom?"[6] when looking at benefits or consequences of doing various practices or using products. Another way of saying this is: "One man's meat is another man's poison."

Living in tune with our constitution goes a long way in alleviating the everyday suffering and distraction we experience. However, this does not mean that we shall live symptom-free or always be blissful. In Tai Situ Rinpoche's *Relative World, Ultimate Mind*, he reminds us that medicine, along with other studies and practices such as art, astrology, geomancy, and language, is useful as a relative means to make our lives more balanced and manageable.[7] By eating well, exercising, relaxing, taking herbs or medical prescriptions, and appreciating our connectedness with the environment, we create a sound biological and psychological state of being which acts as a foundation from which we can embark on or deepen our path toward spiritual awakening. On the journey, as we confront our ignorance, attachment, and aggression we are bound to experience stresses that will be expressed as physical and emotional pain. Perhaps modification of lifestyle will be necessary at that time. But my experience is that if one maintains one's constitutional regimens the spiritual work needed to transform these arising poisons goes more smoothly. One doesn't get trapped in taking symptoms seriously and losing valuable time and energy. This approach is reminiscent of the life of the great Tibetan physician and saint Gampopa. A master physician and student of Tibet's greatest yogi, Milarepa, Gampopa often went through experiences while in spiritual retreat that he assumed to be symptoms of some physical or mental malady that needed fixing. Milarepa's advice to him at those times was to go back into retreat, continue meditating, and not to worry. Inevitably the symptoms passed and Gampopa could see that the symptoms were just the somatic or emotional experience of the Three Poisons. Of course, this does not mean that we should ignore our symptoms and conditions. But it does point to an attitude that I think is important in order for us to ride through the storm fronts that life presents us.

We should view the changes we make to relieve our everyday physical and emotional pain as a means of preparing us for the deeper work needed to bring us awakening to what is our birthright: buddha-nature. If we do not value these deeper, spiritual dimensions of our being and only focus on our healing efforts on stopping our pain, we may feel better temporarily, maybe even until we die at a nice "healthy" old age. But we will have not applied ourselves in a way that will cut through the root of our suffering — our human predicament — in any significant or lasting way. That is why the last chapters of this book are devoted to meditation and spiritual training. For those of you already following a spiritually oriented lifestyle and direction, the physical recommendations contained herein will create a greater sense of mind-body-spirit integration.

It is my fervent hope that you not only feel better from following these recommendations but that you take your newfound energy and focus and aim them towards ends that bring lasting peace and joy to yourself and those around you.

chapter two

NUTRITIONAL PRACTICES

According to Tibetan tradition, the first illness ever recorded was indigestion. The cure was warm water. Thus a causal link between health and what we eat and drink was established.

Correct nutritional practices are a part of the first level of Tibetan medicine, which, as stated in the Introduction, pertains to lifestyle changes. Such practices are considered the least invasive and are, therefore, recommended first or if an illness necessitates greater intervention, in addition to more invasive therapies. Emphasis on lifestyle reminds people of their responsibility regarding disease.

Although it receives more attention in our culture now than previously, the importance of proper nutrition for maintaining good health is still not fully recognized in mainstream society. For the most part, modern clinical nutrition uses the model of the "four basic food groups" and a modern medical model that assesses food for its biochemical composition. The focus is on active ingredients such as vitamins and minerals and the specific effects these substances have on the body. Alternative medical models that use conventional knowledge of biochemistry, as well as focus on the benefits of whole, less processed foods, have become more accepted and have had an impact on conventional medical practices. Still, much of what is recommended in both conventional and alternative health communities is an oversimplified approach to nutrition. Broccoli is good for you. Brown rice and more fiber is what you need. Eggs contain cholesterol, a no-no. What is lacking in this approach is a sensitivity to constitutional variation and how this influences health and illness. For example, there are over a dozen forms of arthritis identified in the Ayurvedic tradition. Depending on the balance of the nyepas due to this condition and the rang-zhin of the person, what is recommended as food, medicine, and therapy will vary.

Perhaps in the early days of medicine in the West, when allopathy was a younger brother to naturopathy and homeopathy, there was a sensitivity to such variation, and the dictum "let your food be your medicine and your medicine, food" was taken seriously. In those times Western culture was more rural, hence agrarian. As we have become urbanized and out of touch with our natural environment, our respect for the elements of which we are a part has been lost. In such a climate allopathic medicine has ascended to a position of almost supreme authority. Losing touch with our natural environment, rhythms of life, and the importance of daily diet and behavior, afflictions such as colds and flus are considered inconveniences in our busy lives. Nature becomes the enemy, and allopathy becomes the hero, with the use of antibiotics, antihistamines, and so forth to keep nature from reclaiming its rightful territory. Ironically, in the end nature does triumph as our symptomology becomes more complex and deep seated. Chronic degenerative disease is the hallmark of modern industrial society. Inevitably this leads to runaway medical costs since interventions need to be more invasive and convalescence prolonged. Although we think that lifespan has increased in modern times due to improved medical care, this is a myth. Improved sanitation has had more impact on health than modern medicine.[1] We have also lowered the infant mortality rates, which accounts for an average longer life expectancy. At the same time, however, we have fewer healthy eighty and ninety year olds; for the most part the senior citizens of our times are more debilitated than in the past. Perhaps we have too readily come to accept this situation as the norm.

The cornerstone of Tibetan medicine and nonconventional health practices today is individual responsibility. Such responsibility should not be considered burdensome. Indeed, being responsible implies being "able" to "respond," to pay attention and reflect on what works and what doesn't work in one's life.

Correct nutritional practices are an obvious place to start. Why? Because selecting, preparing, and eating food is something we do every day and thus plays a major role in how our body functions. Consequently, following good nutritional practices is the first and foremost preventive health-care measure we can take.

Several factors come into play when considering proper nutritional practices.

1. your rang-zhin, or constitutional type
2. your present condition
3. your level of activity (i.e., physical, sedentary)
4. environmental factors

With these basic considerations in mind, we need to look at types of foods, qualities of food and food combinations, as well as when and how we eat.

The following are guidelines to address basic considerations and eating practices, including nutritional recommendations for each of the six constitutional types. At the end of these guidelines, we shall look at factors that indicate whether such dietary practices will work for you.

TASTES

There is more to taste in life than sweet and salty. In Ayurveda and in Oriental healing in general there are five tastes: sweet, sour, pungent (hot), bitter, and salty. When a food does not fall within the properties of these five tastes, it is considered astringent.

Tastes affect the nyepas. They nourish the organs in different ways. Consequently, certain tastes are emphasized in the nutritional recommendations for the different rang-zhins and when there is a specific organ imbalance. The following classifications show which tastes are associated with each of the individual nyepas.

RECOMMENDED TASTES (in order of preference)

LUNG – sweet, salty, sour, pungent

TrIPA – bitter, sweet, astringent

BEKAN – pungent, sour, salty

Combination nyepa-types will work with such information based on the presenting symptoms at any given time. For example, if a LUNG-TrIPA has TrIPA symptoms, the emphasis of the tastes should be those for TrIPA.

Although the food lists presented later in this chapter are extensive, you can expand your dietary practice by considering these taste qualities when selecting foods for your rang-zhin that are not on the lists.

QUANTITIES OF FOOD

Quantity of food here means actual volume. Generally, the amount of solid food you consume should fill two parts, or half, of your stomach. If you were to place your hands together to form a bowl, the amount of food that would fit into your hands would be the amount of solid food you should consume.

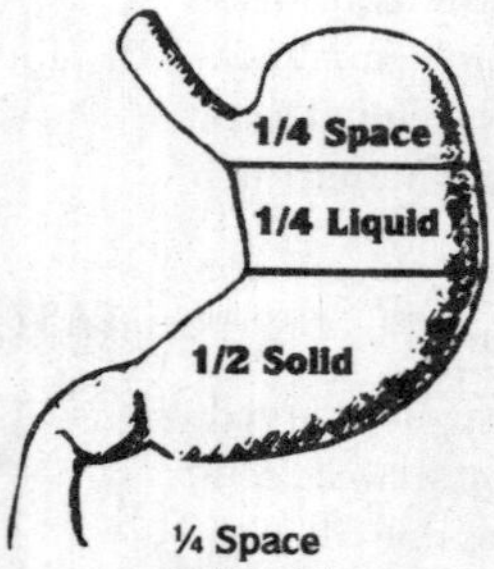

¼ Space
¼ Liquid
½ Solid

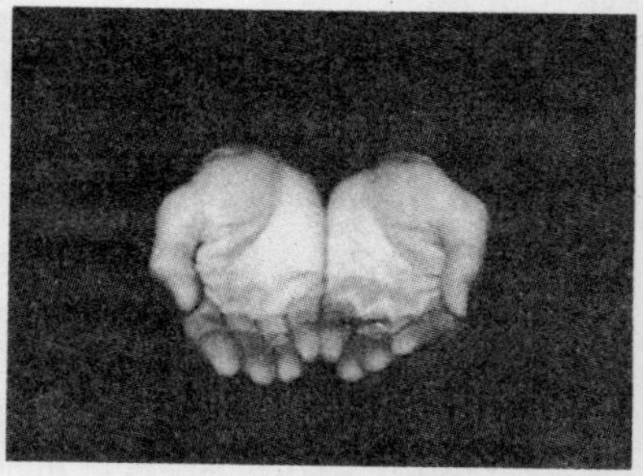

One part of your stomach should be for liquid and one part for space. Space allows for food to mix more easily and thus metabolize more efficiently. If there is less space, foods may putrefy, creating excess BEKAN in the form of mucus.

The quantities of specific foods you should consume depend on where you live and what types of food exist in your region:

1) Foods from wet or humid regions (coastal and tropical) such as seafood and watery fruits and vegetables tend to be heavy and have a tendency to stagnate in the digestive process if overeaten.

2) Vegetables, fruits, and meats from high and dry regions are light and warming and thus can be eaten in more generous portions.

SEASONAL CONSIDERATIONS

During the summer you should follow the above guidelines strictly whereas in winter, because our pores close up and heat is stored, you have more heat to burn more fuel. Thus you can eat more heartily at this time. Chapter 14 of the Ambrosia Heart Tantra elaborates on dietary modifications recommended as the seasons change. These recommendations are based on the taste quality that enhances strength and vigor throughout the passage of time:

> In short, take warm food and drink during monsoon and winter, rough [nourishment] in the spring and cool [food] in early summer and autumn. During the monsoon and winter, take [foods having] the first three flavors [of sourness, saltiness, and sweetness]; in the spring, use the latter three flavors [of bitterness, hotness, and astringency]; and in the autumn, take sweet, bitter, and astringent [foods].[2]

Although not as elaborate, standard macrobiotic recommendations of eating what grows in your climactic region and in season are consistent with Tibetan medicine. Several books on macrobiotics are listed in the Bibliography and are useful to read along with the material on Tibetan medicine and nutrition.

CHEWING

Lino Stanchich, an internationally respected macrobiotic counselor has written an excellent book entitled *The Power Eating Program*, in which he discusses the importance of chewing in the context of nutritional practices.

Chewing affects our metabolism and proper utilization of foods in several ways. First, salivary amylase in our mouths helps break down the starches in grains, vegetables, and fruits into simple sugars. This allows for more efficient use of the energy in carbohydrates. It also allows the stomach and small intestine to focus on protein metabolism without the burden of dealing with starch. Chewing also makes the bones in the skull move more. The temporal lobes of the skull pump as the jaw moves rhythmically up and down. This has a positive effect on the hypothalamus. Thus, endocrine balance and nervous system strength are also enhanced.

Stanchich recommends that people chew each mouthful 75 to 150 times, the latter being preferred. This is especially true for weak or ill individuals. Energy expended in the process of chewing prevents the body from losing heat and energy in the digestive tract and thus aids in the preservation and utilization of metabolic heat, *pho thut* (Tibetan), or *agni* (Sanskrit), in an efficient manner. In addition, chewing slows down the eating process, which allows us to focus on mealtimes as a nutrifying event rather than something that needs to be done while we're on the run.[3]

FOOD SELECTION AND PREPARATION

Cooking is alchemy. You take the elements that have come together as foods in nature and through selection, preparation, and cooking methods create tastes and textures that can be both delightful to the palate and fortification for the body.

The best source for learning how to cook according to constitutional types is Amadea Morningstar's *The Ayurvedic Cookbook* (see Bibliography). The most useful books on food quality, selection, preparation, and cooking techniques are written by macrobiotic authors such as Anna Marie Colbin and Rebecca Wood—to name two outstanding ones (see Bibliography). The following nutritional practice guidelines will be more effective when using these sources for guidance and inspiration.

To date very little has been written about Tibetan cooking. And there is the impression by many who come into contact with Tibetans that all people ate in Tibet was *tsampa* (roasted barley flour), meat, cheese, and Tibetan tea. Although these foods were indeed the common fare for most people, they do not reflect the cuisine of the privileged nor the variety of foods and preparation methods found in the medical tantras. Another question people have about Tibetan diet is that, given the fact that Tibetan culture became Buddhist, why were Tibetans such heavy meat eaters? The answer can be found in an understanding of the terrain of Tibet and a macrobiotic awareness.

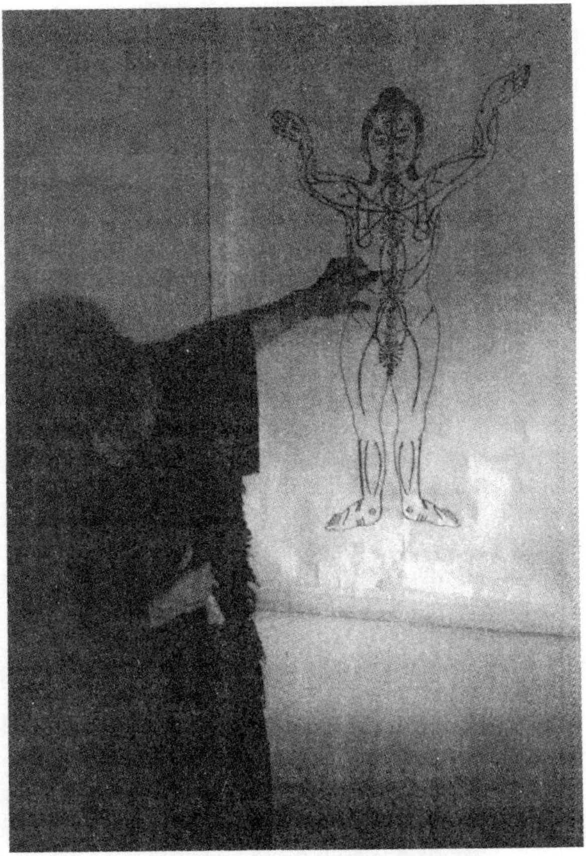

A Tibetan doctor pointing out features of a diagram showing chakras and energy flow. Photograph © by Marica Keegan.

In such a high, dry mountainous climate, there were very few vegetable products, except some grains such as barley and wheat. Also, in a climate where the body is exposed to such extreme natural forces, the consumption of animal food such as dairy and meat products is a way of insulating the body. Unfortunately, this macrobiotic principle has not been well understood by Tibetans who have become refugees in less harsh climates. Such refugees have kept their diet as it was in Tibet, resulting in an increase in digestive, circulatory, and respiratory problems. There are elements of Chinese and Indian cuisine in the nutritional recommendations found in Tibetan medical literature, and to date it is the Ayurvedic cuisine being introduced into the Western world that comes closest to Tibetan cuisine.

When selecting food, it is best to shop at natural food markets and use local sources for the best quality produce. Many of the spices and herbs mentioned below can be found in regular supermarkets. Any additional ingredients that are uncommon or unfamiliar can likely be found in an Oriental grocery. In addition, the Resources at the end of this book will provide you with sources for some specialty items.

FOOD RECOMMENDATIONS FOR THE SIX CONSTITUTIONS

Nutritional Practices for the LUNG-type Constitution

TYPE OF NUTRITION: Because of the variability of physical strength and sensitivity to change, LUNG-types need a diet that is both *warming* and *nourishing*. The diet should be rich in complex carbohydrates and proteins. Cold and raw food should be kept to a minimum.

TIMES TO EAT: Breakfast should be close to dawn and be rich and hearty. The noontime meal should be light, perhaps a soup or light pasta dish. Dinner should be near dusk and be a nourishing, high-protein meal. It is important to be as consistent as possible in keeping regular times for meals.

GRAINS (about 50 percent of the diet)

RECOMMENDED	OCCASIONAL	NOT RECOMMENDED
amaranth	corn	buckwheat
barley		dry oats (like granola and mueslis)
brown rice		
cooked oats		regular white rice
millet		white bread
quinoa		
wheat		
white basmati rice		

PROTEIN (approximately 20 percent of the diet)

LEGUMES:		
adzuki beans	none	Chinese red beans
Anasazi beans		red lentils
black beans		split peas
brown lentils		
garbanzo beans		
kidney beans		
lima beans		
mung beans		
pinto beans		
soybeans		
tempeh		
tofu		

ANIMAL FOODS

cheese	beef	goat
eggs	duck	pork
fish (all types)	fresh butter	
old ghee	fresh cow's milk	
old butter (unsalted)	fresh dried meat	
poultry (all types)	mutton	
whey	rabbit	
	yogurt	

NUTS AND SEEDS

cashew	almond	none
flaxseed	chestnut	
linseed	coconut	
pumpkin	hazelnut	
sesame		
sunflower		
walnut		

VEGETABLES (cooked only)

RECOMMENDED	OCCASIONAL	NOT RECOMMENDED
angelica root	beets	cabbage (raw, generally)
arrowroot	brussels sprouts	lettuce (raw)
broccoli	collard greens	burdock
carrots	eggplant	dandelion greens
cilantro	ginger	bok choy
globe artichoke	green pepper	
onions	hot pepper	
peas	kale	
potato	lettuce	
red cabbage	mushrooms	
sea vegetables	mustard greens	
spinach	parsnips	
sweet corn	turnips	
sweet potatoe		
tomatoes		
winter squashes		

FRUITS (room temperature or cooked)

RECOMMENDED	OCCASIONAL	NOT RECOMMENDED
mango	blueberry	apricot
apple	cherry	cantaloupe
banana	grape	cranberry
grapefruit	peach	dried fruit
pineapple	pear	lemon
orange	plum	watermelon
papaya	strawberry	pomegranate

OILS, SALTS, AND CONDIMENTS

RECOMMENDED	OCCASIONAL	NOT RECOMMENDED
garlic butter	corn oil	mustard oil
ghee	safflower oil	
ginger butter	sunflower oil	
miso		
old butter		
olive oil		
peanut oil		
salt (sea, rock, red, and black)		
sesame oil		
tamari		
umeboshi		

BEVERAGES

RECOMMENDED	OCCASIONAL	NOT RECOMMENDED
cow's milk	wine	black tea
wine		coffee
warm water		cold water
spicy, warm teas (e.g., ginger)		hard liquor

HERBS AND SPICES

RECOMMENDED	OCCASIONAL	NOT RECOMMENDED
angelica	chili	white sugar
anise	coriander	
aquilaria	pippali	
asfoetida	shitavari	
cardamom		
cinnamon		
clove		
cumin		
fennel		
fenugreek		
garlic		
ginger		
jaguri, ghur		
nutmeg		
onion		
raw sugar		
Solomon's seal		
stinging nettle		
terminalia chebula		

Nutritional Practices for the TrIPA-type Constitution

TYPE OF NUTRITION: TrIPA-type persons should generally have a diet that is cooling and a bit more bland than for LUNG or BEKAN. Of the six types of rang-zhin, these people have the more intense cravings for strong-tasting foods and beverages, such as coffee, chili, hot spice, rich meats, and alcohol—which usually aggravate their health problems. Emphasis should be on simple carbohydrates, including some raw foods in appropriate seasons and times. These people have the hardest time maintaining a regimen because they do not like to be told what to do. Relaxation at mealtimes is useful to slow down their sometimes frenetic pace.

TIMES TO EAT: Breakfast should be light or like a small snack. The noontime meal should be the main meal of the day since digestive fire will be particularly strong. A late evening dinner—up until about midnight—is fine, providing digestive fire is strong. Juice or light fasting is OK for TrIPA-types. Be aware that such people can get quite irritable if meals are not forthcoming. A tendency to overeat in such circumstances should be noted and avoided.

GRAINS (approximately 25 percent of the diet)

RECOMMENDED	OCCASIONAL	NOT RECOMMENDED
buckwheat	barley (toasted)	amaranth
corn	oats	brown rice
millet		rye
quinoa		
tapioca		
wheat		
white basmati		
white rice		
white noodles		

PROTEIN (approximately 20 percent of the diet)

LEGUMES:

adzuki beans	chana	Chinese red beans
Anasazi beans	lima beans	red lentils
black beans	tofu	soybeans
brown lentils		tempeh
dahl		
garbanzo beans		
kidney beans		
mung beans		
pinto beans		

ANIMAL FOODS (generally should be kept to minimum)

buffalo	fresh cow butter	beef
cow's milk	fresh goat butter	fish
fresh ghee	pork	lamb
goat's milk	skimmed cow milk	mutton
rabbit		poultry
		shellfish

*(**NOTE:** The hot TRIPA-type, that is with symptoms of diarrhea, migraines, and fevers, should avoid animal products altogether.)*

NUTS AND SEEDS

none	pumpkin	almond
	sunflower	cashew
		chestnut
		coconut
		flaxseed
		hazelnut
		peanut
		sesame
		walnut

VEGETABLES (at least 50 percent of the diet)

RECOMMENDED	OCCASIONAL	NOT RECOMMENDED
asparagus	beet	avocado
bok choy	chard	bamboo shoots
broccoli	cilantro	chili
brussels sprouts	green pepper	eggplant
burdock	Jerusalem artichoke	garlic
cabbage	potato	ginger
carrot	raw spinach	globe artichoke
cauliflower	rutabaga	hot pepper
celery	sea vegetables	mushrooms
collard greens	sweet corn	mustard greens
cucumber		onion
dandelion greens		radish
green beans		sauerkraut
kale		tomato
lettuce		turnip
parsley		water chestnut
parsnip		
red cabbage		
spinach		
turnip greens		
winter squashes		
yam		
zucchini		

FRUITS

RECOMMENDED	OCCASIONAL	NOT RECOMMENDED
barberry	apple	apricot
cantaloupe	banana	cranberry
melons	blueberry	lemon
peach	cherry	lime
pear	grape	
	grapefruit	
	pineapple	
	plum	
	raisins	
	strawberry	

OILS, SALTS, AND CONDIMENTS

RECOMMENDED	OCCASIONAL	NOT RECOMMENDED
fresh butter	corn oil	old butter
ghee	safflower oil	miso
	sunflower oil	mustard oil
	sea salt	olive oil
		peanut oil
		salt (black and red)
		sesame oil
		tamari

	RECOMMENDED	OCCASIONAL	NOT RECOMMENDED
BEVERAGES	water cooling herbal teas (e.g., mint)	skim milk	beer black tea coffee hard liquor wine
HERBS AND SPICES	barberry cucumber seed dandelion ephedra gentian gota kola gugul hibiscus licorice raisins red sandalwood rhododendron rose senica safflower saffron shilajit terminalia belerica terminalia chebula tumeric white sandalwood	cinnamon coriander	

Nutritional Practices for the BEKAN-type Constitution

TYPE OF NUTRITION: BEKAN-types need a warming but light diet that emphasizes light-quality proteins. Very little raw or cold food should be consumed. Eating foods as fresh as possible is also important since overly processed, frozen, or leftover foods can produce BEKAN symptoms such as excessive mucus and a clogged lymph system.

TIMES TO EAT: Breakfast should be eaten between 7 A.M. and 9 A.M., no later. Such people do not need a midday meal, although a very light meal is acceptable. Dinner or the last meal of the day should be eaten between 8 P.M. and 11 P.M.; again the emphasis should be on a light, protein-rich meal. BEKAN-types are encouraged to do routine fasting.

GRAINS (approximately 20 to 25 percent of the diet)

RECOMMENDED	OCCASIONAL	NOT RECOMMENDED
barley	brown rice (with ginger and jaguri)	corn
oats	buckwheat (one year old)	buckwheat (fresh)
white basmati rice	regular white rice	
quinoa	toasted millet	
	wheat	

PROTEIN (approximately 20 to 25 percent of the diet)

Legumes:

RECOMMENDED	OCCASIONAL	NOT RECOMMENDED
dahl	chana	adzuki beans
split peas	brown lentils	Anasazi beans
	mung beans	Chinese red beans
		garbanzo beans
		kidney beans
		lima beans
		pinto beans
		red lentils
		soybeans
		tofu

ANIMAL FOODS

RECOMMENDED	OCCASIONAL	NOT RECOMMENDED
buffalo	fresh cheese (e.g., paneer, farmer)	beef
cheese	mutton (boiled with asfoetida, ginger, and whey)	frozen, roasted, or uncooked meat
fish (all)		goat
aged dry meat		pork
aged butter		
poultry (all)		
rabbit		

NUTS AND SEEDS

RECOMMENDED	OCCASIONAL	NOT RECOMMENDED
none	pumpkin	almond
	sesame (black)	cashew
	sunflower	chestnut
		coconut
		flaxseed
		hazelnut
		linseed
		peanut
		walnut

VEGETABLES (approximately 35 percent of the diet—cooked only)

RECOMMENDED	OCCASIONAL	NOT RECOMMENDED
angelica	arrowroot	(any raw)
bamboo shoots	bok choy	broccoli
celery	burdock	brussels sprouts
chili	cabbage	collard greens

	RECOMMENDED	OCCASIONAL	NOT RECOMMENDED
	daikon	cauliflower	cucumber
	garlic	cilantro	green beans
	ginger	dandelion greens	kale
	green pepper	eggplant	peas
	hot pepper	globe artichoke	potato
	mushrooms	lettuce	squashes
	onion	mustard greens	sweet potato
	rutabaga	parsnip	
	sorrel leaves	sauerkraut	
	tomato	water chestnut	
	turnip		
	young radish		
FRUITS			
	pomegranate	grapes	apricot
	raisins	lemon	banana
	tamarind	lime	blueberry
		orange	cantaloupe
		peach	cherry
		pear	melons
		strawberry	pineapple
			plum
OILS, SALTS, AND CONDIMENTS			
	salt (black)	ghee	fats, generally
	safflower oil	old butter	corn oil
		peanut oil	miso
		sesame oil	mustard oil
		sunflower oil	olive oil
		tamari	sea salt
BEVERAGES			
	beer	black tea	cold water
	warm water	boiled water	hard liquor
		spicy teas	
		coffee	
		cow's milk (warm with spices)	
		wine	
HERBS AND SPICES			
	asfoetida	tumeric	
	ashwagandha		
	black pepper		
	cardamom		
	cinnamon		

RECOMMENDED	OCCASIONAL	NOT RECOMMENDED
clove		
cumin		
fennel		
fenugreek		
garlic		
ginger		
licorice		
pippali		
raisins		
sesame		

Combination Nyepa Constitutions

What follows are the nutritional practice recommendations for those whose constitutions have two fairly equally dominant nyepas: LUNG-TrIPA, LUNG-BEKAN, and TrIPA-BEKAN. Unlike the single-nyepa dominated constitutions, a rang-zhin dominated by two nyepas is indicated in Chapter 1 by having two nyepas whose overall scores are about the same or where the dominance of one over another is marginal. In fact, most people will find that they are classified as combination nyepa constitutions.

In the process of following the nutritional guidelines in the combination rang-zhin chart that follows, you may find that symptoms arise, indicating that the balance of your rang-zhin may be skewed too much in an undesired direction. Again, look at the Chapter "Self-Evaluation," focusing on the section that gives details of symptoms and the nyepa associated with them. Once you have identified the nyepa of your constitution being aggravated, for a period of time follow the single-nyepa nutritional program for that particular nyepa. For example, if you are LUNG-TrIPA or LUNG-BEKAN and you start experiencing gas, bloating, constipation, mental worry, or other LUNG symptoms, for a period of time eat in accordance with the LUNG nutritional recommendation charts. If you are feeling nauseous and have some diarrhea, your eyes are more sensitive to light, or you are more critical or angry towards others, these are TrIPA symptoms. In this case if you are LUNG-TrIPA or TrIPA-BEKAN, eat more in accordance with the TrIPA nutritional program recommendations. Excess mucus, lethargy, sleepiness, and other BEKAN-type symptoms should tell you that in a rang-zhin that is LUNG-BEKAN or TrIPA-BEKAN that BEKAN is out of balance; in this case, for a period of time focus on the BEKAN nutritional recommendations until symptoms subside.

In brief, when symptoms arise, for whatever period of time is needed:

- LUNG-TrIPA or TrIPA-LUNG people with LUNG symptoms should eat from the LUNG list.

- LUNG-TrIPA or TrIPA-LUNG people with TrIPA symptoms should eat from the TrIPA list.
- LUNG-BEKAN or BEKAN-LUNG people with LUNG symptoms should eat from the LUNG list.
- LUNG-BEKAN or BEKAN-LUNG people with BEKAN symptoms should eat from the BEKAN list.
- TrIPA-BEKAN or BEKAN-TrIPA people with TrIPA symptoms should eat from the TrIPA list.
- TrIPA-BEKAN or BEKAN-TrIPA people with BEKAN symptoms should eat from the BEKAN list.

In general **Combination Types** should concentrate on the following foods:

	(LUNG-TrIPA)	(TrIPA-BEKAN)	(LUNG-BEKAN)
GRAINS			
	amaranth	barley	barley
	barley	corn	oats
	brown rice	millet	toasted millet
	cooked oats	quinoa	white basmati
	millet	tapioca	
	quinoa	wheat	
	wheat	white basmati	
	white basmati	white noodle	
PROTEIN			
	Legumes:		
	adzuki beans	adzuki beans	dahl
	Anasazi beans	Anasazi beans	split peas
	black beans	black beans	
	brown lentils	brown lentils	
	chana	chana	
	dahl	dahl	
	garbanzo beans	garbanzo beans	
	kidney beans	kidney beans	
	lima beans	mung beans	
	mung beans	pinto beans	
	pinto beans		
	tempeh		
	tofu		
ANIMAL FOODS			
	butter	buffalo	beef (boiled with asfoetida, ginger, and black salt)
	cow's milk	cow's milk	

	(LUNG-TrIPA)	(TrIPA-BEKAN)	(LUNG-BEKAN)
	eggs fish (all) poultry (all) rabbit	ghee goat meat goat's milk rabbit	buffalo cheese fish (all, cooked with brown sesame seeds) fresh dried meat poultry (all, cooked with brown sesame seeds) yogurt
NUTS AND SEEDS	cashew flaxseed linseed pumpkin sesame sunflower walnut	pumpkin sunflower	none
VEGETABLES:	*(steamed/raw)* angelica arrowroot beet broccoli carrot cilantro globe artichoke green pepper onion peas potato red cabbage sea vegetables spinach sweet corn sweet potato tomato winter squashes	asparagus bok choy broccoli brussels sprout burdock cabbage carrot cauliflower celery cilantro collard greens cucumber dandelion greens green beans kale lettuce parsley peas potato red cabbage spinach turnip greens winter squashes yam zucchini	*(cooked only)* bamboo shoots celery daikon eggplant garlic ginger globe artichoke green pepper lettuce mushrooms mustard greens onion parsnip radish rutabaga tomato turnip

	(LUNG-TrIPA)	(TrIPA-BEKAN)	(LUNG-BEKAN)
FRUITS	apple banana blueberry cherry grapefruit orange pineapple plum strawberry	barberry cantaloupe grape melons peach pear strawberry	grape peach pear pomegranate raisins strawberry tamarind
OILS, SALTS, AND CONDIMENTS	corn oil garlic butter ginger butter ghee miso olive oil peanut oil salts (all) safflower oil sesame oil sunflower oil tamari	fresh butter ghee sunflower oil (no salt)	salt (black) safflower oil sunflower oil
BEVERAGES	cow's milk warm water	water	warm water spicy teas
HERBS AND SPICES	anise aquilaria cinnamon clove coriander cumin fennel fenugreek ginger jaguri nutmeg onion sesame Solomon's seal terminalia chebula	embilica officinalis gota kola gugul hibiscus licorice raisins red rose red sandalwood safflower shilajit shitavari terminalia belerica terminalia chebula tumeric yellow rose	angelica asfoetida ashwaghanda black pepper cardamom cinnamon clove cumin fennel fenugreek garlic ginger sesame

FOOD COMBINING

The following guidelines for combining foods come from the medical tantras and the teaching of macrobiotics in which I have counseled people over the years.

The transcontinental and international shipment of foods has created opportunities to eat foods from different climates and cultures. This may appeal to our gourmet palates, but it puts stress on our bodies. Regional cuisines arose out of necessity. However, while learning to use what food sources were available in the immediate environment, people developed an understanding that such practices also helped in promoting good health. Every indigenous culture has daily, festive, and medicinal cuisines. To utilize such foods out of context, that is out of season in different climates, in the wrong circumstances, or mixed with inappropriate foods creates digestive instability and threatens health. In the future this will be exacerbated by proposed genetic engineering practices whereby, for example, carrots may be infused with banana DNA to make them grow larger and sweeter. Indeed, combining food on the genetic level will make the literature on the benefits and actions of foods on the body virtually meaningless.

Still, while the marketplace drives the food industry in this precarious direction, there is a growing number of people who want quality organic foods grown in their regions. As regards combining foods, it is advised to eat *regionally* and *in season.* Such foods reflect the influences of the climate and thus help the body in adapting to the climate. It is advisable to know what type of climate you live in (temperate, arctic, mountain, tropical, and so forth), learn which foods grow in that region, and select such foods from local sources or from places where the climate and seasonal patterns are the same.

The following general rules for combining foods will help in the proper assimilation of what you eat.

1. **Grains plus legumes, seeds, or nuts** create *whole proteins.* However, people usually use equal amounts or more of legumes, seeds, or nuts to grain. At any meal, when grain is

offered, protein-rich foods should be about one-half or less of the size of the grain portion.

2. **Avoid eating animal and vegetable protein-rich foods together.** Combinations such as meat plus beans, nuts, or seeds, such as a hamburger plus baked beans, are difficult to digest. Your body has enzymes designed to break down animal *or* vegetable proteins at any one time. If eaten together, your body does not know which enzymes to add to the stomach, so it will send in none. The result is putrification and gas.
3. **When eating meat, reduce your quantity of grain and eat more vegetables.**
4. **Eat melon-type fruit by themselves.** Melon is the fastest-digesting food there is. If eaten as a dessert or with a meal, your body will choose to digest it and leave everything else to be digested in a much less efficient manner. Melons can be eaten as a snack or an appetizer about twenty minutes before a meal. Using melon as an appetizer is particularly useful for TrIPA-types.
5. **Fruit as dessert is best in cooked or stewed form** (compote, applesauce, fruit crumbles or cobblers). Especially if having a meal with legumes as the main protein, wait approximately twenty minutes for dessert. Avoid raw fruit as dessert; instead, eat raw fruit as a snack by itself or as an appetizer.

There are also more specific food combinations that are generally not advised. These are:

- Curds or yogurt mixed with new wine
- Fish and milk or milk products (e.g., British-style poaching)
- Milk and walnuts (and other nuts) cooked together
- Fruit juice and milk (e.g., juice and cereal with milk at breakfast)
- Eggs and fish (e.g., tuna salads with mayonnaise)
- Yogurt and peas and molasses
- Mushrooms and mustard
- Chicken and yogurt or curds (although the spices of tandoori style are useful here)
- Honey and oil
- Peaches combined with other fruits

It is also said that if one food discolors another in the process of cooking, such a combination is toxic. (This does not apply to dye effects of beets or purple cabbage.)

Another form of food combination to avoid is eating meals too close together so that a previous meal is not fully digested. The second chapter of the *Gyud-Zhi* says, "The quantity of food taken in the morning should be such that one is able to digest it by the afternoon, and the quantity taken in the evening such that one can digest it before dawn."[4] Food taken at the right time in the right quantities will strengthen pho thut, or digestive fire, and help to prevent disease. If you feel full or heavy with food or you have no immediate urge to eat, wait.

Although Amadea Morningstar's *The Ayurvedic Cookbook* avoids combinations mentioned above, it does combine LUNG, TRIPA, and BEKAN foods. Knowing how to use spices and understanding what quantity or proportion works best, the author is able to provide a wide range of culinary opportunities that will not conflict with the dietary regimens listed above.

FOOD QUALITY AND SPECIAL FOOD GROUPS

When Ayurveda was developed and the medical tantras written, food was unadulterated. Thus the effects of foods in various states and preparations were known. Beyond the specific recommendations for constitutional types and specific health conditions, people were discouraged from eating food that was burnt, rotten, or in any way spoiled. Such rules obviously still apply.

Food should be as fresh as possible. Of leftovers, Dr. Yeshe Donden says,

> Leftovers after many days will overpower the digestive fires of the stomach. In general, it is said that after twenty-four hours any food is stale. Even in a refrigerator, the cold causes it to come into this class."[5]

Such food will increase BEKAN, thus mucus and congestion, creating tiredness. Basically it is devitalized. Consequently, other than filling the stomach, it has little benefit. This, no doubt, also applies to overly processed foods and prepared frozen meals. Of freezing, Dr. Donden says that only raw meat is not harmful after being frozen.[6]

Food selection based on quality and freshness has become increasingly complex in modern times. What is most commonly available in the marketplace of the modern world bears little resemblance to foods available eighty, let alone hundreds to thousands of years ago.

The abuse of fertilizers, pesticides, and hybridization have created grains, fruits, and vegetables that are low in nutritional value. Demineralized, overplanted soil also leaves fruits and vegetables weak and demineralized. Even that which is called "fresh" has often been preserved by chemicals (such as sulfur dioxide), petroleum-based waxes, or through gamma radiation. Such practices have arisen not because of their nutritional benefits but because of economics.

Most domesticated animals to be used for meat supplies are treated inhumanely. Poor living conditions, chemicalized food sources, and antibiotics used to either stave off infection or to bloat the animals for more mass create animals that are weak and diseased. In the case of dairy products, it is not an uncommon practice to have small computer chips placed underneath the cows' skin to monitor hormone levels. When the levels drop (as would naturally be the case when mothers stop nursing their young), the cows are given additional hormones to increase milk production. This often leads to teat infections, which in turn are taken care of by antibiotics. Residues of these antibiotics remain in the milk and may be the cause of colic and other problems commonly experienced by young children fed cow milk. In *Diet for a New America*, John Robbins talks about such issues, not only from a nutritional standpoint but also from a moral point of view. In fact, he states the greatest travesty of the current time may be the inhumanity we show other species of life.[7] Stephen Gagne's *Energetics of Foods* and Annemarie Colbin's *Food and Healing* also discuss these issues (see Bibliography). Not long ago, I heard from news reports that if the most recent liver transplant from a baboon to a human is successful, the market for available livers will increase and baboons will be bred for their organs. Another example of this exploitation attitude is the slaughtering of black bears in China, solely for the purpose of removing bile from the gallbladders—bile being renowned for its medicinal properties and even recognized in Tibetan pharmacopeia. At the same time, there are vegetable alternatives such as saffron, which is recommended by Tibetan doctors to create similar effects. As we become more sensitive to the interdependence of species in maintaining global harmony, it behooves us to search for effective alternatives to the unnecessary slaughter of another species, which may have short-term benefits for the few but will inevitably create more suffering for the many.

When I first met Tibetans who were just settling in the United States, they found it almost incomprehensible that any government would allow its food supply to become poisoned. Starry-eyed with the abundance of America, their assumption was that if a food was in one of those amazing supermarkets it must be good. No doubt this is equally true of the average consumer who is not taught nutritional principles or does not have access to information about how the food industry has come to be driven by profit rather than health considerations.

A good example of this situation occurred while I was working with a Tibetan doctor. One Tibetan treatment that is periodically used to renutrify a person who is weak is milk enemas. The doctor had decided to administer such an enema to a friend and asked me to go to the supermarket to get a carton of milk. However, after I explained the homogenization process, whereby fat molecules are reduced to the size of water molecules in order to enhance shelf life but with questionable repercussions to health, he decided that maybe it wasn't such a good idea after all.

Thus when putting the nutritional recommendations into practice, you should not only adhere to the quantity of the suggested regimen but you should also pay attention to quality. Meats that are organically grown are recommended. Dairy products should be chosen with equal scrutiny and should be consumed in accordance with Ayurvedic principles. Ice-cold milk, cheese, and ice cream are considered heavy, cold, and mucus-forming. However, warm milk, yogurt, and cheeses cooked into vegetables and with spices can be enjoyed according to constitution and condition without the physical side effects often attributed to dairy products.

Select organic grains and legumes as the staples of the diet. Vegetables and fruits should also be organic. However, since these cannot be stored like grains and legumes, and their availability is more sporadic, fresh fruits and vegetables from the supermarkets can be used. To nullify the effects of fertilizers and pesticides, Dr. Hazel Parcells, a well-known and respected American naturopath recommends the following procedures. These methods have been tested and confirmed as effective by the Sierra States University School of Nutrition.[8]

Food Cleansing Formula One is a formula for foods that have been irradiated. To find out if your foods have been irradiated, you will have to speak to the produce, meat, and dairy (for eggs) supervisors of your local markets.

Add one tablespoon of baking soda to every gallon of water used. Soak the irradiated products in this formula for the times listed in the chart below. Then soak them in fresh cold water for an additional ten minutes to eliminate the soda taste.

Food Cleansing Formula Two is for foods that you know are not organically grown. As most markets like to advertise that products are organic, it is reasonable to assume that anything not labeled this way is not organic.

Add one-half teaspoon of plain, old-fashioned chlorine bleach (e.g., Clorox) to every gallon of cold water used. This will not affect the taste of your foods, nor will it cause damage in any way. After the prescribed amount of time soaked in the formula, place the foods in cold water and soak them for an additional ten minutes. The soaking time for this formula and Formula One are as follows:

Leafy Vegetables.................10–15 minutes
Root Vegetables..................15–30 minutes
Thin-skinned Berries.........10–15 minutes
Heavy-skinned Fruits.........15–30 minutes
Eggs....................................20–30 minutes
Meat per pound (thawed)...5–10 minutes[9]

Of such methods, Dr. Parcells says that they will make vegetables and fruits crisper and taste better as well as increase their shelf life. They will also eliminate the toxic residues within the animal foods mentioned.

OTHER ENVIRONMENTAL CONSIDERATIONS: Water and Air

At the beginning of this chapter, the story was told of how warm water was the medicine used for the first illness of mankind: indigestion. Indeed, even in modern times, the importance of ample water as a part of daily liquid intake is acknowledged in conventional and alternative health circles alike. However, what quality of water is necessary to derive health benefits is widely debated.

According to medical and Buddhist tantric literature, there exists a pure water of almost unworldly nature. It has eight special qualities; it is (1) extremely cool, (2) fresh, (3) tasty, (4) soft, (5) clear, (6) free from impurity, (7) soothing to the stomach, and (8) clears the throat.[10] Waters of the Ganges and other holy water sources such as the Chalice Well of Glastonbury are considered to be such waters. All other waters are compared to these.

The *Gyud-Zhi* classifies water as being beneficial according to the following order:

1. Rain water
2. Melted snow water
3. River water
4. Spring water
5. Well water
6. Sea water
7. Forest water[11]

Of the most beneficial water, rain water, the text reads

> . . . although rain water is vitalizing, refreshing, pleasing to the stomach, thin, satisfying, stimulating to the intellect, of indistinct taste, savory, light, cool and nectar-like, touched by the sun, moon, and wind while falling, its wholesomeness or unwholesomeness depends largely upon the time and place.[12]

To test the purity of such, the text goes on,

> [The rain water is to] be collected in a bowl and mixed with unstained rice pap. If the mixture does not become discolored or putrid, the rain water is wholesome.[13]

Following the 1991 Gulf War, it was reported that several months after the igniting of the oil fields of Kuwait, the snow was a blackish color in the Himalayas. Thus even in the purest of areas of the world, it is neither the time nor place to find water of pure quality. Acid rain is a documented problem throughout the world. Where there is no modern-day sanitary awareness or practices, microorganisms that lead to severe gastrointestinal distress abound. And in areas where water sources are monitored, petro-chemical and chlorine levels create other kinds of physiological distress.

It is a necessity of the times that the water we ingest requires special attention. Certified pure, bottled water or some form of in-home purification system is advisable. The three most common systems for purification are distillation, use of a carbon filter, and reverse osmosis. In virtually every major city in the modern world, it is possible to find sources for such purification systems. Experts on these different systems espouse theirs as the best choice; and readers are encouraged to do their own research of the various systems before making a selection. Although such practices are not mentioned in the tantras, in order to have water available that possesses the qualities of water mentioned in the tantras purification seems necessary.

Obviously, the quality of water and air influences everything that grows. Although in-home purification of both is possible, we cannot monitor the water and air that our plants are grown in. And although we can choose not to drink water other than that which comes from our homes or is bottled, unless we wear a gas mask we have to breathe the air that surrounds us.

As the oxygen level on the planet diminishes with increasing carbon monoxide and ozone depletion, the oxygen level in plants and animals also diminishes. With such diminished levels of this element, our food supplies are not as life-giving as in the past; and since oxygen is important to our bodily health, this profoundly affects our vitality and immunity. In the Chinese medical classic *Yellow Emperor's Classic of Internal Medicine*, the relationship between breathing and digestion is emphasized. According to this text, there are subtle energy channels from the lungs to the stomach that allow *chi*, or life force, to stimulate digestion in the stomach. If the lungs are blocked or there is coughing or breathing is affected, the stomach is equally affected.[14] In the literature of India's Hatha Yoga tradition (much of which was incorporated into Buddhist practice, particularly in retreat situations), it is even said that if the right sinus is blocked, resulting in labored or uneven breathing, one should refrain from eating.

Although we can probably only affect the overall quality of air through political and/or economic means, we can follow a few simple rules when utilizing the air and oxygen available. These rules pertain to eating and proper assimilation:

1. Eat fresh foods rather than old or processed foods.
2. Do not eat on the run.
3. Chew well.
4. Be relaxed and breathe calmly while eating.
5. Eat in a well-ventilated space whenever possible.

Other considerations are to get appropriate exercise and select clothes of natural fibers that allow the pores of your body to breathe. This is especially important for undergarments.

SUPPLEMENTATION: Vitamins, Herbs, and Super Foods

Although supplementation to food was once considered to be necessary only for the infirm, weak, or diseased, given our current biological condition, the state of our food supply, and the conditions in which we live today, such supplementation seems to be essential to proper nutrition. It must be understood that when we speak of supplements we are distinguishing them from medicines. As an adjunct to sound nutrition, supplements are preventive rather than curative in nature. Although supplements can help restore body balance so that the body is no longer a host to disease, to rely solely upon supplementation for cure of medical symptoms is to run the risk of overestimating their benefits.

When suffering from a disease condition, it is always best to use your preventive health-care knowledge along with sound medical information and guidance.

When selecting herbs and vitamins, principles of Tibetan pharmacology are useful. In Tibetan medicine, constitution and daily condition are always considered when it comes to the selection of herbs and nutritive substances. To ensure that these will be metabolized in the body and create the desired effect, Tibetan doctors utilize Chinese principles for creating herbal remedies. Never is a single herb prescribed alone. All herbs are considered to have side effects when used alone, and both in Tibetan and Indian Ayurveda as well as Chinese herbology, side effects are considered signs of inappropriate medicine. Rather, herbs are combined; in Tibetan medicine, a minimum of five are usually considered best. Such compounds consist of the main herb, the one you are trying to get to a certain part of the body to create an effect; herbs to alert the body to changes; herbs to clean the pathways of the body for the main herb to get to its final destination; and herbs to act as carriers for the main herb(s). The point is to prepare the body to accept the desired substance for maximum assimilation and utilization, with no side effects. Some of the more progressive Western herbologists practice herbology with such an understanding. However, a good deal of popular herbology extols the virtues of this herb and that herb without taking such subtleties into account. To some extent, it is the progressive researchers into vitamin supplementation and therapy who have grasped principles comparable to those of Tibetans and Orientals more than herbalists have. For proper absorption and utilization, vitamins and minerals are chelated, are micellinized, given more digestible coatings. Some are even time-released.

Whether you take prescribed supplements or ones that you think are good for you, to be beneficial they need to comply with the conditions discussed above; they must be in keeping with your rang-zhin, your present physical and mental condition; be of good quality and easily and efficiently absorbed; and be taken in a timely, appropriate manner and in keeping with a sound nutritional program.

It is not always possible to adhere to such criteria. Perhaps we do not know of a good herbalist, naturopath, or Ayurvedic or Chinese health practitioner. And of the over-the-counter type supplements, all claim to be better than others. How can you confidently select the best and most effective ones?

What follows is an excellent Tibetan medical means of testing which supplements are best for you. This test is very simple and can be done in your own home. It was shown to me during a Tibetan medicine program under the guidance of Dr. Lobsang Rapgay.

Tibetan Urine Testing for Supplements and Medicines

This technique will only work with substances that are in powder form, including foods, herbs, vitamins, and medicines, be they allopathic, herbal, and so forth. It will not work with gelatin capsules, oils, or liquids.

Upon rising, use a clean jar to collect the midstream of your first morning urine, dispensing with the first and last parts of your urine, which have the largest amount of toxins and waste products. The midstream urine has semimetabolized substances from foods, vitamins, and so forth and is considered the cleanest. For a woman, it is best that this test is not done during menstruation.

To do this test you will need the following:

1. a small pot for heating the urine
2. shallow white or unpatterned clean bowls in which the urine will be pored
3. a mortar and pestle, useful for substances that need crushing (Powders will, of course, not need further crushing.)

Procedure:

1. Take each supplement to be tested and crush with the pestle in the mortar if necessary. If in capsule form, open and remove the gelatin capsule. Do each supplement or substance separately and place the powder on a piece of clean paper in front of one of the bowls. Be sure to label the powder so that you know which substance you are testing in a given bowl. Wash the mortar and pestle in between substances to avoid contamination due to mixing.

2. Pour the urine from your jar into the pot and heat it slowly on the stove until it just begins to steam—a bit higher than body temperature.
3. Using one bowl for each substance to be tested, pour the urine from the pot into the bowls so that it is about three-fourths of an inch deep. This means that you can only test as many supplements and medicines as the amount of your urine supply will accommodate.
4. Take a pinch of the substance before one bowl and drop it into the center of the urine in the bowl.
5. Observe the rate of dispersion and whether part of the powder sinks or not.

A supplement or substance is good for your body if, when you drop the powder on the surface of the urine, it spreads rapidly across the entire sample and none of it sinks.

A supplement or substance is not useful for your body if, when you drop it on the surface of the urine, it sits in the middle without spreading and/or starts to sink.

A supplement or substance is neither good nor bad if it spreads slowly, does not spread out over the whole sample but stays more contained, and then some of it sinks. In this case such a substance may be good at some times and not at other times. It deserves retesting at a later date, but at present it is doing little to benefit your body.

There are also cases in which some of the powder spreads very fast and part of it sinks. This indicates that you may need to take each one of the mixture's ingredients and test it separately.

6. Repeat this test for each powder in front of each bowl.

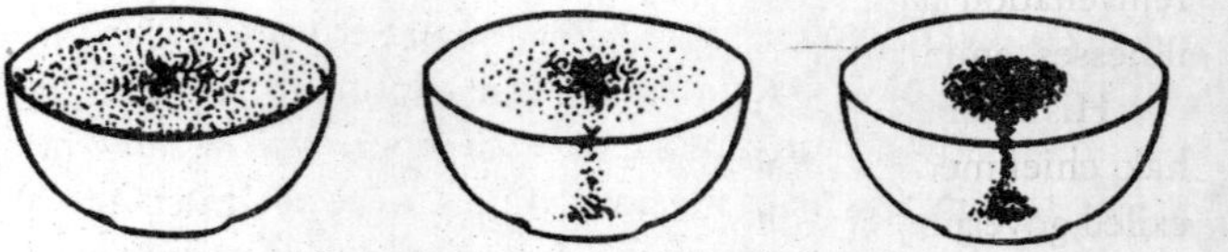

Good **Fair** **Not Good**

Since results of this test are dependent on your current state of health more than your rang-zhin, it is best to test supplements and medicines about every three weeks to see how your body is handling them if you are planning on taking them for a prolonged period of time. It is possible that as your condition changes, substances you are taking are no longer needed and to continue taking them may have adverse effects. It is also possible that your needs will change in accordance with changes in seasons, climates, and other conditions. Hence, the usefulness of this test.

This is a good method to use at home when pulse diagnosis cannot be done. To my mind, it is more objective than kinesiology, although with oil-based substances, gel capsules, and liquids, kinesiology may be the next best low-tech or home method to employ.

Such a method also eliminates our subjective desires to see certain substances work better than others. Sometimes we think that natural or herbal substances are superior to processed, allopathic medicines. I have seen many clients shocked to find out that their allopathic medicines were better for them than some of their herbal supplements. The body knows what it needs, and its natural intelligence is generally more accepting than our mental concepts.

TIBETAN PRECIOUS PILLS

Tibetan Precious Pills are used in different ways to restore and promote vitality. They are used as a monthly supplements for rejuvenation and preventive health care, as medicines for specific illnesses, and in a spiritual context.

His Holiness the Dalai Lama entrusted Dr. Tenzin Choedhak, chief medical officer of the Tibetan Medical Center at the exiled government seat of the Dalai Lama in Dharamsala, India, to start producing these pills. The main ingredient of these pills is tsothel, "a purified and detoxified mercury powder with a sulfur base."[15] Detoxified metals such as mercury are called *basmas* in Sanskrit. Tibetans are renowned for their meticulous attention in making basmas. Precious and heavy metals are heated until they oxidize, resulting in substances that are no longer toxic and travel deep into the body for the purpose of rebuilding body strength. To these oxidized precious and heavy metals are added herbs and other vegetation, as well as sacred materials, the origin of which is known only to the pharmacologists, herbalists, and spiritual teachers authorized to create and utilize them.

Precious Pills traditionally come wrapped in small colored silk pouches, the color of which identifies them. They are taken in a ritualistic fashion, late at night and usually on auspicious days such as full or new moons, and accompanied by prayers. Precautions and instructions on how to make a given pill more effective are usually given. However, in medical emergencies, Precious Pills can be taken on an as-needed basis in order to take advantage of the power they have.

The following excerpts indicate the Precious Pills' ingredients, actions on the body, rituals, and precautions. *These are deep acting and long lasting.* Although the urine test could be done to see if one of these pills is suitable for you, it is best to take them on the advice of a Tibetan doctor or tantric master. The text of the first three pills mentioned is from the Tibetan Medical and Astro Institute. The description of the last pill, Precious Old Turquoise 25, is from Kunphen Tibetan Medical Hall and Clinic in Kathmandu.

Rinchen Tso-Tru Dhashel *(Precious Purified Moon Crystal)*

> This Precious Rinchen Tso-Tru Dhashel has been compounded from about fifty different ingredients following the exact formula developed by the renowned fifteenth-century Tibetan scholar and physician Surkhar Nyam-Nyi Dorjee.
>
> This precious pill is an antidote; it purifies and helps with the circulation of blood, it heals stomach ulcers, liver ailments; it stops severe pains and ailments caused by sudden changes in diet and climate. It heals hidden fevers and chronic ailments after a fever, when one cannot eat well and there is loss of hair and loss of strength and clarity of the teeth and nails. It is excellent for combatting infections and inflammations. It also heals ailments caused by excess of diet and alcohol. It is a good tonic for dark, thin persons of weak constitution. This pill clears the senses and restores

the memory. It treats inflammations of the chest, including persistent cough with blood and phlegm discharges as well as breathing problems. It also combats retention of water in the body. When one is in good health, this pill will help to better the health, prolong one's life, and it is a rejuvenating agent.

Some of the ingredients in this pill are gold, silver, copper, brass, lead, and bronze, which are purified of their toxic effects before being mixed with other herbal ingredients such as gynachum forresti (schitr), saussaure lappa (Clarke), commiphora mukul (Angl), strychonos nux-vomica (linn), myristica fragrans (Houtt) and eugenia caryophyllata (thumb). Many sacred pills and the precious Ngochu-tsothel are also added to this pill.

Detailed instructions for taking this medicine is mentioned in the medical texts, but the following prescription will be sufficient. This pill should be taken on an auspicious date, though at the time of an illness, this pill is taken when needed. Before retiring to bed, take a clean, unbroken cup and put a crushed pill in this cup, adding a small amount of hot water, and cover the cup with a clean cloth. Early next morning, take the ring finger of the right hand and stir the mixture in the cup while repeating the mantra of the Medicine Buddha—TA-YA-THA OM BAY-KAHN-DZE BAY-KAHN-DZE MAHA BAY-KAHN-DZE RAH-DZA SAH-MOOD-GAH-TAY SO-HA. Drink this mixture followed by a cup of hot water. Retire in bed with this thick coverings for about an hour so that the body perspires.

On the day this medicine is taken and if possible, a couple of days thereafter, refrain from taking meat, eggs, fish, uncooked grains, garlic, onions, alcohol, sour foods, and drinks. Raw vegetables and fruit, old and pungent food should be refrained also. One should not undertake strenuous exercises nor sleep in the day, and one should refrain from sexual intercourse and cold baths. No other medications should be taken on the day this pill is taken.

It is most important that this pill should not be exposed to direct sun or lamp. It should be prepared and taken in dim light.

Although the preparation of the following two Precious Pills varies from that of Rinchen Tso-Tru Dhashel, many of the ingredients are the same. Rather than list all of the ingredients, I shall only list their actions and for whom they are most appropriate. The precautions for all of them are virtually identical and will therefore be omitted in the descriptions.

Rinchen Mangjor Chenmo *(The Great Precious Accumulation Pill)*

The effects of the Great Precious Accumulation Pill is to pacify the 404 main ailments caused by the disorders of the blood, bile, mucus, and wind of the body. It also heals old wounds of the head, chest, limbs, swelling of the throat, leprosy, and epidemics. It protects one from evil spirits who cause illnesses. There is no ailment this pill cannot cure. If one is in good health, this pill will help to better the health and prolong one's life. It is especially effective to treat food poisons, animal and insect bites, rabies, and plant poisons. It also helps treat old and hidden ailments, fever and when one passes blood from the bowels or from the mouth due to severe illness.

If one is ill, this pill can be taken at the moment required without considerations to the above conditions.

Rinchen Ratna Samphel *(Precious Wish Fulfilling Jewel)*

The Rinchen Ratna Samphel, or the Precious Wish Fulfilling Jewel, is an antidote. It combats food poison; plant, insect, and animal poisons; chemical poison and poison from the sun rays etc. It is beneficial for all strokes and paralysis, for trembling and numbness in the body, for lame and dislocated limbs, for all types of nerve disorders. It also combats persistent urination due to nerve disorder, helps those who have difficulty in opening and closing the eyelids, heals deafness, loss of smell, loss of body sensation, and loss of the control of saliva. It is good for controlling high blood pressure, heart ailments, pulmonary TB, blood clots, ulcers in the body, and primary cancer cases. It is also extremely beneficial for relieving pain in advanced cancer patients, and it cures sudden ailments caused by different spirits.

Obtaining this Precious Pill is like obtaining a precious jewel from the King of Medicines.

Rinchen Yu Nying 25 *(Precious Old Turquoise 25)*

This Precious Pill is made according to the method developed by Pon Tsang Zana. It consists of 25 ingredients. It is prepared from old turquoise, coral, pearl which are purified of their toxic contents. Other constituents are purified iron fillings, asphaitum, crocus satirus linn, muschus moschiferous (musk), the three myrobalans without seeds, two types of sandalwood, euqunia caryphyllata (thumb), saxicus pasumensis marg, and addatoda Vasica. Much prayers are recited during and after the pills are made.

Old turquoise is a special pill. It is detoxicating and of a cool nature. It is good for all liver ailments. It cures liver pain, enlargement of the liver, loss of weight due to liver ailment, and when there are destruction of the nerves of the liver. It also helps to release the pressure on the upper part of the body, relieves stiff neck, headaches due to blood pressure, nose bleeding, bloodshot eyes, pain under the armpits, loss of appetite due to stomach disorder. It treats damaged liver which is caused by over consumption of alcohol and food poisoning.

On the day this pill is taken refrain from sour food and beverages, raw vegetables and fruits, garlic, onion, rancid food; and one should not indulge in strenuous physical activities.

The Resources at the back of the book will provide you with addresses to get more information about and to order these Precious Pills.

DIGESTIVE FIRE

We have talked about the importance of food quantity and quality, taste, chewing, breathing, and relaxation in connection with the process of digestion. We shall now discuss metabolic heat, or digestive fire, known as *pho thut* (Sanskrit: *agni)*. The Sanskrit term *agni* refers to a number of different types of heat processes in the body. However, the Tibetan term *pho thut* relates specifically to digestive fire.

Let us assume that you have learned to eat the right foods in appropriate quantities. You chew well and try to breathe and relax while you eat. All of these facilitate good digestion. However, what if you generally feel tired and lethargic after eating? Perhaps you have chronic low back pain and still have persistent intestinal symptoms like gas, or dry or watery bowel movements. You may even notice allergy-like symptoms and lower resistance in the spring and fall. All of these symptoms can be the result of excessive or insufficient digestive fire.

In *Tibetan Medicine and Other Holistic Health-Care*, Dr. Tom Dummer quotes Dr. Pema Dorje in a 1985 article written in the Tibetan Medical Institute Newsletter:

> Digestive fire is like a machine; diets are the raw materials and bodily elements are the products. No one can expect a good product from a defective machine even if the raw materials are of good quality. Similarly, weak digestion will serve the body with no healthy elements or tissues. For example, one can find a weak and skinny son in a wealthy family which can afford the best foods available, while on the other hand, strong healthy people can be found in poor families who live on simple food. What is the reason for this contradiction? A person should have good digestion so that food eaten will be assimilated by the body. It is said in the Tibetan medical texts that almost all of the chronic and internal diseases originate from indigestion. So it is very important to maintain digestive fire.[16]

Disturbance of digestive fire in the various nyepa-type constitutions is primarily due to poor nutritional habits; eating foods not in keeping with your constitution, excessively or insufficiently, and not following other good dietary practices all contribute to this condition. Beyond this, the tendency of people in Western cultures to consume excessively high amounts of stale, overly processed, fatty foods, drink iced beverages with meals, and overeat all lead to the disturbance of digestive fire.

Excessive digestive fire, or pho thut, arises from the overconsumption of meat and the use of coarse spices. Spices can inflame pho thut; meat demands the digestion to burn hotter to metabolize the meat. Belching, diarrhea, excessive perspiration, thirst, and general mental overexcitability are signs of excessive pho thut.[17] Generally, the reduction of such foods to an appropriate level for a given constitution will ameliorate this situation. If such habits go on for too long, however, they can push the body too far, in which case pho thut is extinguished. High pho thut then becomes low pho thut. And for the most part, low pho thut is the problem that most people face who have digestive fire difficulties.

In *The Ayurvedic Cookbook*, Amadea Morningstar suggests eating smaller meals, and drinking lime or lemon water and a mild ginger tea to help rekindle pho thut. Often times the herb and spice combinations in Ayurvedic and Tibetan cuisine are precisely for that purpose. The use of spices like cumin, coriander, and fennel in cooking or in their seed form in equal amounts as a tea are considered a means to "stimulate and tonify"[18] pho thut. She also suggests that there are different formulas for LUNG, TrIPA, and BEKAN, utilizing fresh gingerroot as a base that can be taken before eating:

For LUNG—grated ginger + pinch of salt
For TrIPA—grated ginger + pinch of raw sugar
For BEKAN—grated ginger alone[19]

Dr. Lobsang Rapgay suggests that the macrobiotic miso-based soup with some fresh ginger is an excellent starter for LUNG. For TrIPA, start with a small green salad. BEKAN can use *trikatu* (a mixture of equal amounts of powdered ginger, cayenne, and black pepper) as an appetizer to stimulate pho thut. Trikatu is sprinkled onto a quarter teaspoon of honey and taken ten minutes prior to eating.[20] The *Gyud-Zhi* recommends the use of a small amount of wine after a meal to stimulate digestive fire.[21] In Indian Ayurveda, there is a wine made of grapes and herbs called *draksha* which is excellent for this purpose. Also, Tibetans have a custom of drinking boiled water served hot ten to fifteen minutes after a meal. Experience has shown me that this latter custom is an excellent digestive aid.

Of the remedies mentioned, the miso soup for LUNG, light green salad for TrIPA, and Amadea Morningstar's suggestion of light ginger tea for BEKAN seem to be the most acceptable in daily nutritional intake. They can increase and maintain pho thut.

Wine at the end of a meal should be considered curative rather than routine, thus used in cases where the digestion is weak. On the other hand, drinking hot water after a meal suits all constitutions as a daily practice.

ASSESSING NUTRITIONAL PROGRAMS

To know if a diet is good for you, you should adhere to the selected nutritional program for at least three to six weeks. However, before making changes in your diet in accordance with your rang-zhin, you should assess your metabolic heat, or pho thut, based on the symptoms discussed. If there are symptoms, try to correct this situation by following some of the recommendations provided before proceeding with a dietary change.

According to naturopathic and homeopathic traditions, every twenty-one days your body goes through a natural healing crisis, whereby your body is adjusting to the nutritional input of this time period. Going through one or two of these cycles with a new nutritional program ensures that your body is on a new track. Take your pulse and check your urine daily during this time. Observe any symptoms. If your condition remains stable and your energy constant, the diet is good for you.

Dr. Yeshe Donden's words best sum up the importance that Tibetan medicine places on proper nutritional practices:

> If you partake of food and drink well, your body and life will be sustained well, whereby you will live long. If you do not know how to eat and drink properly—if these are insufficient, excessive, or perverse—disease will be produced, and your body and life will be adventitiously over-powered. Hence, those who want happiness should value skill in eating and drinking.[22]

chapter three

EXERCISE

The Tibetans I have encountered over the years are very hard working and resourceful. No matter what their professional training may be, they are prepared to roll up their sleeves when the task demands.

Because their lifestyle includes farming, nomadic herding, and making crafts involving physical labor, there was and still is plenty of exercise in daily Tibetan life. Tibetans also have a tradition of enjoying competitive sports, especially contests of strength and horsemanship. Yet, there does not seem to be much specific information on exercise in the available translated material on Tibetan medicine.

In the Ambrosia Heart Tantra, or *Gyud-Zhi*, those who have BEKAN-type complaints (such as lots of mucus and congestion, lethargy), are generally strong, or tend to eat a lot of rich, oily food are encouraged to exercise in winter and spring. After such exercise they are advised to do the following:

> [Afterwards] one should [rub oil on the body, and then when perspiration has appeared], apply [lentil flour all over the skin]. [Finally], dry [the body by rubbing it with a towel]. This rids [the body of excessive] phlegm, aids the digestion of fat, [gives] a clear complexion, and is the best [means] for strengthening the limbs [and making them supple].[1]

It has been my experience that rubbing sesame oil into the skin before exercise, followed by a lentil or chickpea flour rub to pull out the toxins that get attracted into the oil from the exercise, is an excellent regimen to practice. Rubbing sesame oil over the body before exercise is especially recommended for LUNG-type constitutions.

Exercise is also considered an integral aspect in the Tibetan treatment of mental problems as elucidated in texts on Tibetan psychiatric practices presented in Terry Clifford's *Tibetan Buddhist Medicine and Psychiatry*.[2]

Beyond consideration of specific medical conditions, perhaps Dr. Yeshe Donden's answer to a question on jogging best summarizes the Tibetan medical view on the relation of exercise to good health:

> *Question:* Do you think that joggers are wasting their time?
>
> *Answer:* Jogging can be helpful for the body if proper diet is enacted simultaneously because it makes your body more healthy, firm, strong. Still, the main thing is food; for instance, you cannot operate a car without gas. If you do not eat well and go out and exercise, it will ruin your body, but if you eat well and exercise, you will be in good health and strong.[3]

In our more sedentary culture, people often exercise for enjoyment rather than as part of work or a specific curative process. In all three scenarios, however, we should emphasize exercise that best suits different constitutional types. In the cases of manual labor and exercises that are recommended for healing, it makes sense for people to understand what is best for their particular constitution so that they do not overtax themselves and can work more effectively or can enhance the healing process. In this book it is neither possible nor appropriate to discuss specific occupational exercise or healing regimens. Rather, the intention of this chapter is to help readers understand approaches they should take in some common forms of exercise and sport, and to introduce them to some of the beneficial exercise processes available in the Tibetan culture. Although not every sport or type of exercise is discussed, once you understand how to approach an exercise process or sport in accordance with your rang-zhin, the guidelines in this chapter can be applied to the exercise or sport of your choice.

Because this chapter focuses on exercise in relationship to the individual nyepas, those whose constitutions are dominated by two nyepas should shift emphasis in exercise based on diet, symptoms they are experiencing, and the season.

EXERCISE FOR THE LUNG CONSTITUTION

LUNG-type constitutions do best with gentle and consistent exercise programs. The gentle movements of yoga and tai chi are excellent. Exercise that encourages chaotic breathing or makes you constantly out of breath should be avoided. It is also important for LUNG-types to build up stamina. This should be done gradually and consistently—to counteract the LUNG tendency to be intense and do to much, then collapse.

Before sports and exercise in general, rub your body with sesame oil, especially the joints. Begin whatever form of exercise you do with a good, gentle stretching series. Although jogging, running-type sports, and walking are all fine, be careful not to jar the joints of the body. This is one reason for avoiding high-impact aerobics (not to mention the fact that it creates erratic breathing). Quality, appropriate footwear is recommended. Bodybuilding is fine, so long as the body is oiled and the build up of weights is gradual. Inversion machines and yogic postures that invert the body are also excellent for LUNG-types since they help to redirect circulation through the colon and thus have a rejuvenating effect.

Avoid exercise in chaotic environments or adverse weather conditions, where you feel physically or emotionally uncomfortable. A stable, serene atmosphere where there are few distracting influences is recommended. Also, consistent eating habits will facilitate benefit from exercise.

EXERCISE FOR THE TrIPA CONSTITUTION

Because of good stamina, these athletic types can enjoy most forms of exercise. TrIPA-types are the most competitive of all the different constitutions. The downside of this characteristic is that competitive situations can accentuate their tendency towards aggression. This includes competing with themselves where they can overtax their capacities by creating unrealistic expectations. Such aggression towards the self or others can create more stress than benefit from exercise.

Because TrIPA-types tend to be overdoers they should avoid midday runs or exercise in extreme heat. Sweating should be kept to a minimum. Exercise that emphasizes spinal flexibility is excellent. Swimming and exercising near water (even ice skating) or where it is possible to gaze out over vast distances helps to dissipate TrIPA intensity. In general, TrIPA-types need to balance exercise with *quality relaxation*—being able to let go.

TrIPA-types should be sure to replenish the body with lots of fluids but avoid ice-cold drinks during or after exercise. Overall, the emphasis in exercise should be on pleasure and relaxation rather than competition.

EXERCISE FOR THE BEKAN CONSTITUTION

In Tibetan medical literature, BEKAN-type complaints are addressed with exercise. The reason is that with BEKAN-types and BEKAN-related complaints, there is a tendency to become lethargic and overweight. BEKAN-types need to be aroused, woken up.

These people are encouraged to work out. Exercise and sports that have unpredictable movements like basketball, soccer, and racket sports help to stimulate the BEKAN physique. It is also helpful to encourage circulatory and lymphatic stimulation. Mini-trampolines or rebounders are excellent for this purpose. In addition, because of the denseness of their bodies and gracefulness such types exhibit while in motion, they can benefit from aerobics. Breaking a sweat from exercise is good. The oil and flour procedure mentioned at the beginning of this chapter is helpful to clear away BEKAN-type discharges that create heaviness, i.e., mucus, excess oiliness. The oil used can be a sesame-ginger combination or some kind of stimulating liniment.

The challenge for BEKAN-types is getting into the mood to exercise. Once they start, they will see the benefits.

SEASONAL CONSIDERATIONS

In Ayurvedic tradition, people are encouraged to exercise in accordance with seasonal influences as well as individual constitutional variations. Generally speaking, spring and fall are times when one can exercise to full capacity. Summer heat exhausts energy fast so it is best to avoid becoming overheated during this season. Setting out to break a sweat at this time is ill-advised since it could lead to prolonged exhaustion; and excessive sweating weakens the heart. In winter you should exercose at one-half of your capacity to ensure that you build up energy and heat rather than exhaust it. At this time of year too much exercise can deplete metabolic heat and energy, leaving the body vulnerable to disease.

★ ★ ★

What follows are brief histories and descriptions of exercise forms that have come from the Tibetan martial arts tradition or monastic settings. The illustrations will show you how they appear so you can consider whether or not such types of movement appeal to you.

These exercise series are suitable for all constitutions. I can personally vouch for their benefits in everyday life and stress management. Addresses for more information and where to train in these techniques is listed in the Resources section.

TIBETAN TAI CHI AND CHI KUNG

I first encountered Tibetan tai chi in 1987 when staying with friends in Albuquerque, New Mexico. I had daily morning exercise routines I had done for some time. One morning when I was doing my exercises, my friend was doing his tai chi. I had seen the classical Chinese tai chi form and had never been particularly attracted to it. Yet this system seemed different, more meditative, animal-like, and low to the ground. It was quite a powerful experience just to watch it.

Soon after this incident, I had the good fortune of meeting Liu Siong and his wife, Marilyn, at their Garuda School of Tibet Tai Chi and Chuan Fa. Liu Siong was half Chinese and half Dutch by birth. He was raised in Indonesia and was sent by his family to the Shaolin Temple in China to summer-long training for fifteen years. Only a handful of students were selected to learn the Tibetan form of tai chi, the first movement of which tradition holds came from the First Dalai Lama. When students of the yang, or more conventional tai chi, came near the practice area, those performing the Tibetan form were instructed to stop their practice because it was considered secret.

After the Japanese invasion and Communist takeover of China, Shaolin became a museum and tourist attraction rather than a place for spiritual and martial arts training. Only a few people knowledgeable in the Tibetan forms of the martial arts survived, and only Liu Siong received these teachings in their entirety. He then transmitted this knowledge to his wife Marilyn, who, since Liu Siong's passing, has continued to teach.

Tai chi is a way of balancing, regenerating, and storing *chi* in the body. Roughly translated, chi means life force. In Sanskrit the word for this life force is *prana* and in Tibetan, *LUNG*. In this case LUNG is that which keeps the body alive, vibrant, and moving. Tai chi is meditative movement, where body, mind, and breath are harmonized. Tibetan tai chi can be subdivided into four distinct, yet interdependent phases. The first phase of the sequence is a yang, or hard, form, where movement is done while holding one's body tense, like a full-body isotonic. This drives the chi deep into the body. While performing it, one feels as if an attack with iron bars and swords would just bounce off of the aura of energy one projects. This phase is taught last because the body needs to be more settled and balanced before it is truly effective. Thus, in the classroom, this phase is actually called the fourth phase, even though it is really the first in the series of phases one would do to complete the form.

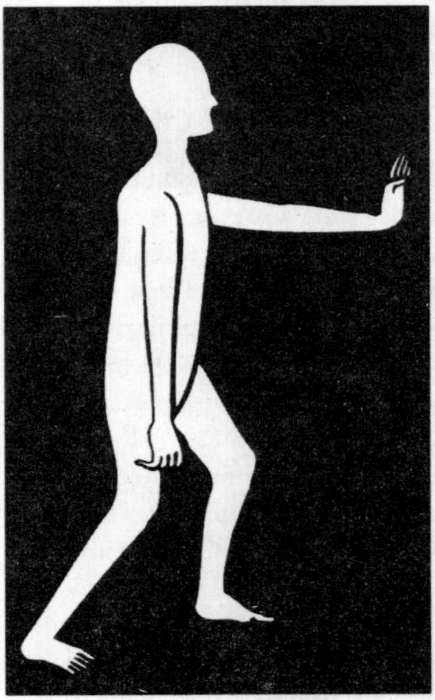

First move, first phase.

What precedes this fourth phase are the first three phases. These have a softer, more yin quality. These phases are taught sequentially, building on the energy and balance created. Each movement has a name of its own such as "stepping over rocks" and "lion goes down the mountain." There are also exercise series to make the tai chi more effective. After learning these softer phases and various other exercises, the yang, or first, part of the series is taught.

My experience in studying and practicing this system is that it is very effective and its benefits are accumulative. The age of students in the classes I attended ranged from under ten to over eighty. All body types benefit, and I have personally observed the elimination of chronic symptoms and illnesses in myself and other practitioners of this gentle martial arts form.

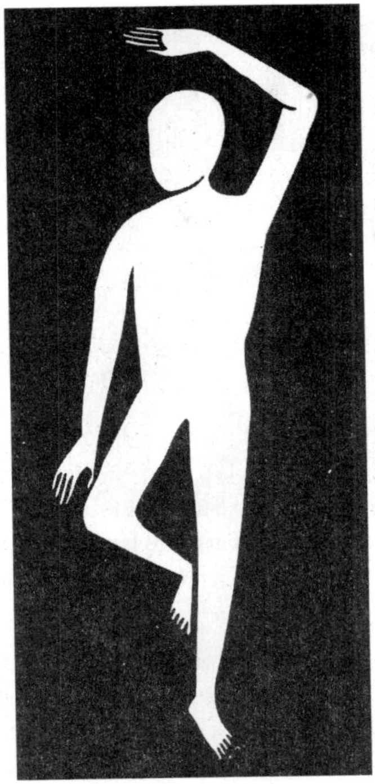

Stepping over rocks.

TIBETAN CHI KUNG

Although similar to many martial art forms of exercise in that there is a mindfulness in the interaction between mind, body, and breath, in *chi kung* the emphasis is on breath and mind with the movements being slightly more passive. The speed and forms of movement are similar to tai chi, but here hand postures, or *mudras*, and the way one visualizes energy and the breath moving are crucial.

For more than ten years, the Western medical community has been interested in chi kung as reports from China tell of its curative effects on heart disease, cancer, and stress-related illnesses. Reoxygenation of the body is probably one aspect of its

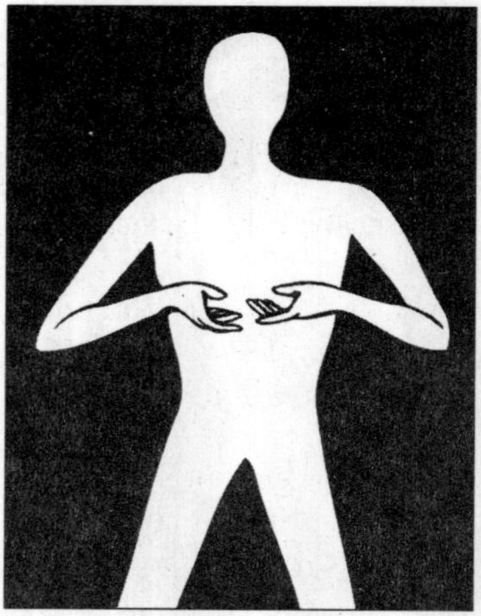

A movement in Tibetan chi kung.

curative power. Another important aspect is the emphasis on mind and body being in sync. Over time, researchers will find that dissociation and denial, where a person cuts themselves off from emotions as a way of anaesthetizing the body, is extremely damaging. Chi kung and other systems of mind-body exercise may be vital ways of bringing people in touch with their emotions, thus bringing them back to life.

For those who want to learn more about Tibetan tai chi and chi kung, see the listing of the Garuda School of Tibetan Tai Chi in the Resources section.

KUM NYE

Kum nye (pronounced koom nyay) has been introduced to Westerners by Tibetan Buddhist master Tarthang Tulku, Rinpoche. It is a system that utilizes the dynamics of stillness, breathing, and self-massage to create a sense of balance and personal mind-body integration. Tarthang Rinpoche learned these exercises from his father, who had learned them in a similar fashion from other Tibetan teachers. Although the exercises that comprise kum nye can be found described in Tibetan medical texts and Buddhist literature over the centuries, kum nye was primarily transmitted orally, from teacher to disciple. Teachers initiating their students in the oral introductory yoga tradition of the *nying-thig tsa-long* (subtle body energy)[4] used the exercises as introductory methods of mind-body integration to facilitate a more balanced spiritual development. Tarthang Rinpoche has taken the liberty of modernizing the system for the purpose of making it more accessible to Western cultures.

Tarthang Rinpoche is an eloquent writer, capable of introducing concepts related to mind, body, and actions in an almost poetic way. Thus it is only fitting to quote him in the explanation of the initial aspects of kum nye and what to expect from practicing them:

> In Kum Nye, there are various ways, including both stillness and movement, to stimulate the flow of feeling and energy which integrates body and mind. We begin by developing stillness of body, breath, and mind. Simply sitting still and relaxing gives us a chance to appreciate feelings of which we are normally unaware. This relaxation is then subtly aided by breathing through both nose and mouth so gently and evenly that we are hardly conscious of inhaling and exhaling at all, a way of breathing which allows us to contact the positive vitality of the throat center.
>
> As the breath becomes calm and quiet, fewer distracting thoughts and images run through the mind, and the whole body becomes alive. Our mental and bodily energies become refreshed and tranquil, like a clear forest pool. We discover a quality of feeling common to body, breath, and mind—a calm, clear, deepening quality—which soothes and massages us deep within. As we relax more, the subtle level of this feeling opens like a lens, letting in more "light" or energy and creating more comprehensive "pictures" of experience.[5]

Self-massage is then added to deepen one's experience of relaxation. Deep relaxation, as Tarthang Rinpoche describes it, goes far beyond our conventional notions of relaxation, which is primarily focused on pleasantly distracting ourselves. In this case, relaxation is shedding old mental and physical patterns and waking up dormant energies so that we can regain our childlike wonder of the world. Again, exercise need not be excessively strenuous or painful to have a positive effect. With our energy moving more freely and relaxed, vitality and strength arise naturally. In Melanie Sachs's description of the benefits of massage, she captures the state of mind emphasized in kum nye: "Gentleness and mindfulness are the attitudes to embrace towards yourself when exercising. Exercise to benefit yourself and others, not out of dissatisfaction for your shape, size, or condition."[6]

The Nyingma Institute under the guidance of Tarthang Tulku, Rinpoche, has published two volumes on kum nye (see Bibliography), as well as exercise audio cassettes. Rinpoche recommends them for young and old alike; it is safe for anyone to practice them, even without a teacher. People who want more information and personal training should contact the Nyingma Institute listed in the Rejuvenative Resources section.

TIBETAN REJUVENATION EXERCISES

In 1989, a friend of mine who was studying Ayurvedic medicine told me about a book he thought would interest me. The book had a rather tabloid title: *Ancient Secrets of the Fountain of Youth*. The author, Peter Kelder, tells of an elderly British officer whose quest it was to find a legendary Tibetan lamasery, reputed for teaching its monks and lamas a way to slow down and reverse aging. The author meets this officer before and four years after he finds the "fountain of youth." Kelder reports amazement in witnessing the transformation of his elderly, somewhat frail friend to a younger looking, robust figure of a man.

This Shangri-la-type story may appeal to some; it did not to me. However, I was curious about the exercises that Kelder describes as the "Five Rites."[7] In his *Inner Power: Secrets from Tibet and the Orient*, Christopher S. Kilham calls them the "Five Tibetans."[8] Having practiced these five exercises now for six years on a daily basis, I am convinced of their power to rejuvenate. In fact, I have been told by friends that I look younger now than I did six years ago.

Many things labeled "Tibetan" are considered esoteric. Because these exercises derive from yoga, some may feel that they will only suit contortionists. But fortunately this is not the case. Tibetan Rejuvenative Exercises—as I call them—are extremely simple to do. Of course, if you have some physical limitations, you may need to modify or omit one or more in the series. In Kelder's edition, the British officer led classes with the elderly and infirmed, with excellent results. In some cases, modification of the exercises was necessary, but with continued practice even these people were able to eventually perform all exercises in accordance with their original descriptions. In any event, whether you are young or elderly, you should be able to build up to twenty-one repetitions of each exercise as recommended. Like many exercise series that have arisen from a more spiritual understanding of our true capacities, Tibetan Rejuvenative Exercises benefit all seven of the constitutional types.

Of these exercises, Christopher Kilham says:

> The Five Tibetans stimulate the chakras and their corresponding nerve plexuses and glands. By balancing the psychic energies of the body-mind, they promote a strong immune defense system, maintaining keenly developed nerve transmission, and establish a balanced hormonal climate. They tone and stretch major muscle groups, creating a strong, flexible physique.[9]

It is best to do these exercises in the morning soon after getting up, although they can be done at any convenient time. To perform twenty-one repetitions of all the exercises takes only ten minutes. They are an excellent way to shake off any morning dullness and are recommended before doing meditation. Thus they promote physical well-being and enhance spiritual practice.

Rejuvenative Exercise #l

The first exercise involves spinning. The dervish tradition of Sufism recognizes the power of such stimulation. In this context, the spinning activates the chakra/endocrine systems. It is the energy activated by the spinning that makes all of the other exercises of this series beneficial.

Rejuvenative Exercise #1: Spinning.

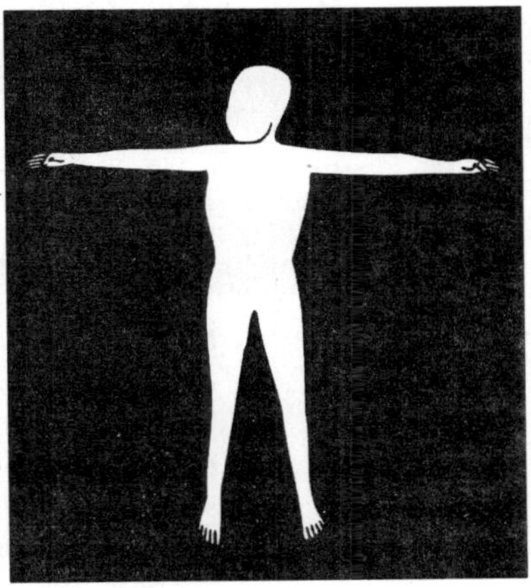

It is natural for a person to feel some dizziness from doing the spinning. That is the sign of a healthy vestibular system. Thus, do not be alarmed. Also, as with all of these exercises, begin slowly. Start with seven spins and gradually work up to twenty-one.

STEP 1: Stand straight and allow your arms to be outstretched with fingers extended, palms downward. Keep your arms at shoulder height—not above, not below. This will help to activate the maximum amount of chi, or life force. Allow your tongue to rest on the roof of your mouth, just behind your teeth. Although this procedure is not specified in the literature, this will permit more cerebro-spinal fluid to move along your spine, enhancing the exercise. It also activates what in Sanskrit is called the *brahma-randra*, the crown point of the skull, which in turn allows more psychic and spiritual energy to enter the body.

To reduce dizziness, before starting to spin focus on a point in front of you. As you complete each spin, let your eyes return to the same point.

Spin at a comfortable rate in a clockwise direction. This means that initially your right arm goes back and your left arm comes forward as you move.

STEP 2: At the end of the spins, rest your hands on your hips. Breathe in through your nose and out through your mouth two to three times. Then lie on your back with your arms to your sides, palms down. This is the position to start Rejuvenative Exercise #2. At the same time, the palm-down position of the hands also lessens the dizziness.

Rejuvenative Exercise #2

It is best to do Exercise #2 through #5 on a cushioned surface, i.e., carpet or exercise mat.

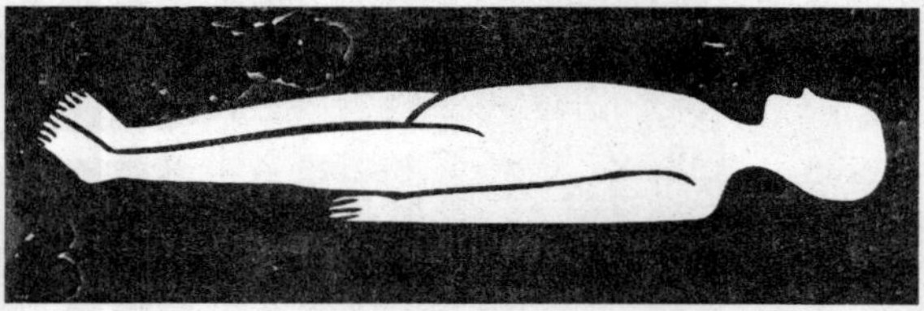

Exercise #2 Step 1.

STEP 1: As described at the end of Exercise #1, for Exercise #2 you begin by lying on your back, your arms to your sides with your palms downward.

STEP 2: As you inhale, simultaneously bring your head off of the ground so that your chin comes towards your chest and raise your legs so that they are perpendicular to the ground. A little beyond perpendicular is fine, but try to keep your legs as straight as possible. (If this is difficult to do, bend your knees to the degree that helps. Over time, your back and abdominal muscles will become strong enough to perform this exercise with straight legs.) Then, exhale and lower your head and legs to the ground, again simultaneously. Allow all of your muscles to relax for a moment and then repeat the exercise. Work up to twenty-one repetitions.

After the spinning of Exercise #1, all of the Rejuvenative Exercises emphasize stretching and bending the spine. In the yogic tradition, this is considered to be rejuvenating. In Exercise #2 you are stretching the cervical and lumbar spine. By lifting the legs, you are also activating what is known as the sacral pump mechanism. This allows for more efficient cerebro-spinal fluid movement through the entire spine. It has a positive effect on the entire nervous system and encourages proper circulation in all internal organs, especially in the abdominal region.

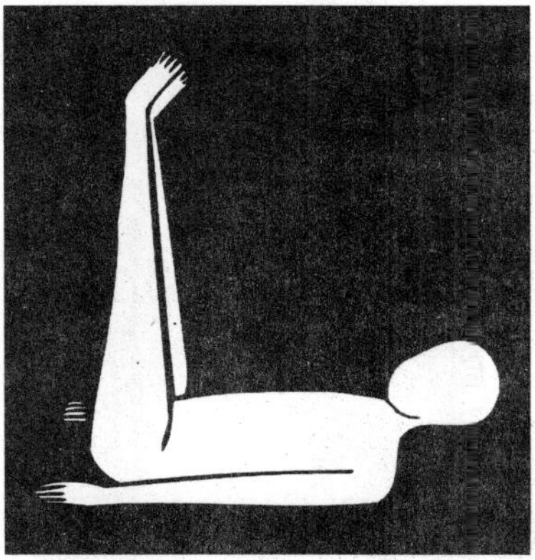

Exercise #2 Step 2.

Rejuvenative Exercise #3

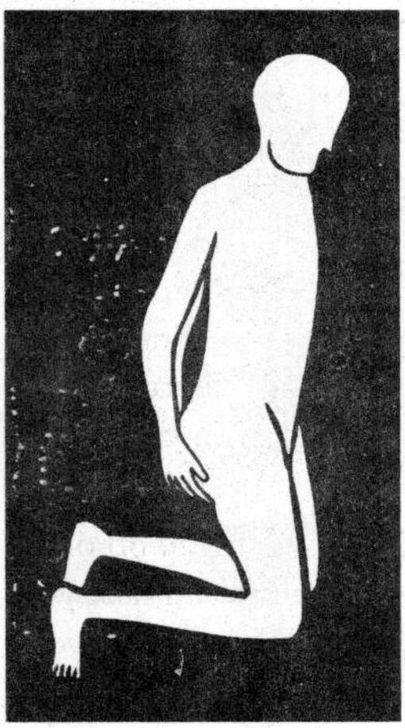

Exercise #3 Step 1.

Step 1: After regaining your breath to a normal, relaxed rhythm from Exercise #2, position yourself so that you are kneeling, your knees about one fist distance apart and your toes curled up. Allow your hands to clutch just below the buttocks on the back of your thighs. Place your chin to your chest.

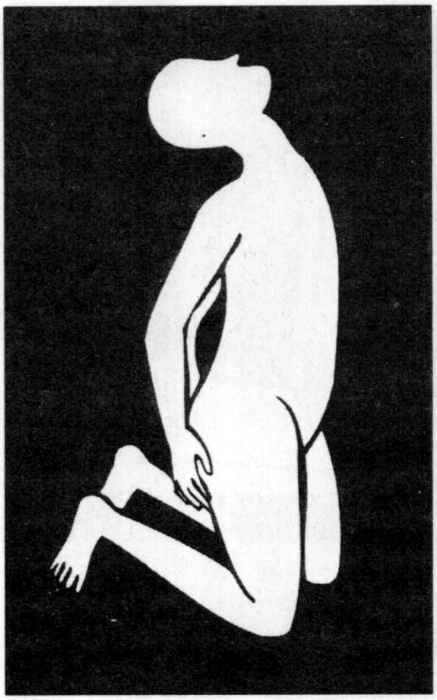

Exercise #3 Step 2.

STEP 2: As you inhale, tilt your head back as far as it will go, lift your chest, and pull your shoulders back so that your upper spine is arched. As you exhale, return your chest and shoulders to a more natural position and allow your chin to once again rest on your chest. Repeat. (Remember to keep your tongue resting on your upper palate.)

This activates the energy vortices, or chakras, and endocrines in the neck and chest: thyroid, parathyroid, and thymus. Arching of the spine stimulates the brachial plexus at the base of the neck, thus strengthening the arms and shoulders and increasing circulation to the lungs, heart, and the chest region.

Rejuvenative Exercise #4

STEP 1: Sit so that your legs are extended out and your feet are about twelve inches apart. Place your arms to your sides so that your hands are palms down on the ground beside your buttocks, your fingers pointing towards your feet. Your chin is, once again, touching the top of your sternum.

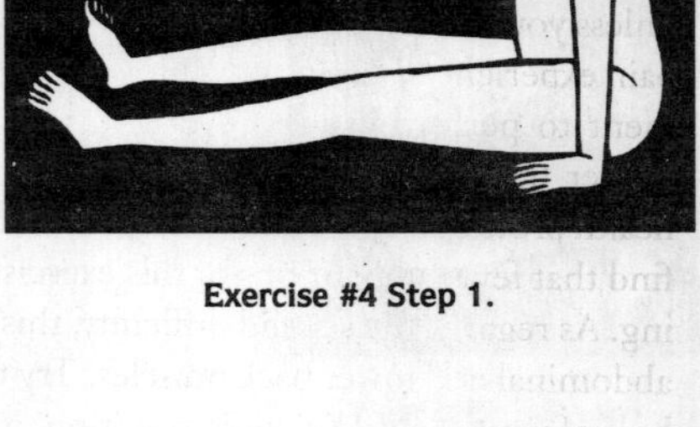

Exercise #4 Step 1.

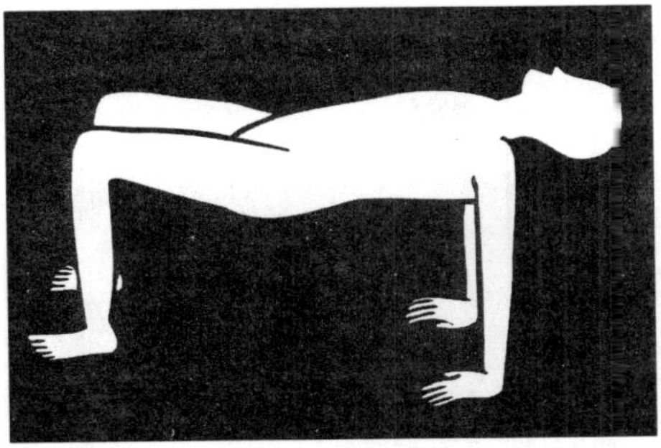

Exercise #4 Step 2.

STEP 2: As you inhale, lift your buttocks off the ground and allow your head to drop back. The final position of this movement should be where your legs are bent at a right angle at the knees with your feet on the ground, your abdomen and chest parallel to the ground, your arms straight, and your head dropped back so that you are looking at what is behind you upside down. (This is similar to the table pose in Hatha Yoga.)

In this posture, hold your breath and tense all of your muscles—your legs, arms, buttocks, abdomen, and chest. As you exhale, relax all of your muscles and allow your body to come down into the original posture as shown in the Step 1 drawing. Repeat the desired number of times, eventually working up to twenty-one.

This is a strenuous posture, and its benefits are great. The abdominal muscles and organs are tonified, the solar plexus region is energized, and the life force is driven deep into the body with the isometric tensing.

It is important to maintain regular and balanced breathing while performing this exercise. If you become winded, pause between repetitions. Two other difficulties that people report in doing this exercise are pains in the shoulders and an inability to bring the torso to the parallel position. Regarding the first, unless you have a specific shoulder or upper arm complaint, the pain experienced during or after is a beneficial structural adjustment to performing the exercise. If such a pain persists for longer than three weeks, however, it is advisable to consult a health professional. People with specific shoulder complaints may find that fewer repetitions of this exercise promotes faster healing. As regards the second difficulty, this often arises from weak abdominal and lower back muscles. Try to lift yourself up to the best of your ability. In yogic tradition, it is said that if you visualize yourself moving into the perfect position while performing a given posture, movement, or exercise to the best of your ability, slowly you will find that you improve. *This advice is applicable to all forms of exercise.*

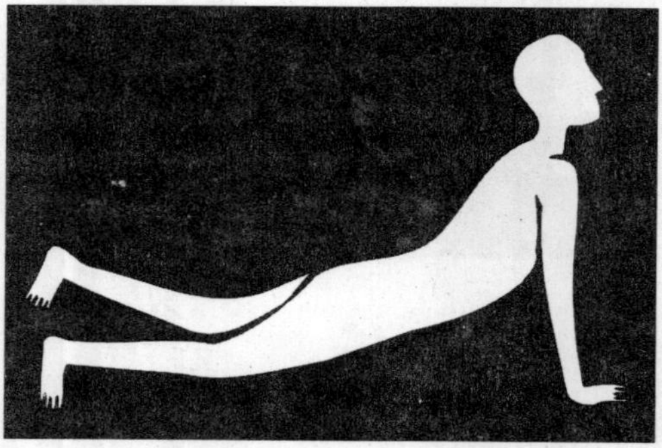

Exercise #5 Step 1. (When modified, knees rest on ground.)

Rejuvenative Exercise #5

This exercise is akin to the dog posture in Hatha Yoga, only more dynamic.

STEP 1: Place yourself in a push-up type position with your hands and feet both about two feet apart from each other. Allow your toes to be curled and your back to sag so that you are looking forward. Your arms and legs should be straight. You are actually holding your body off the ground with your hands and toes. Do not allow the fronts of your legs or hips to touch the ground.

As you inhale, lower your head and raise your behind so that you are looking between your own legs. Your behind should be higher than any other part of your body. As you exhale, lower yourself down into the original position. Repeat.

The arching of the entire spine in this exercise helps the immune system and rejuvenates the nerves in the spine. You are also strengthening both your arms and legs.

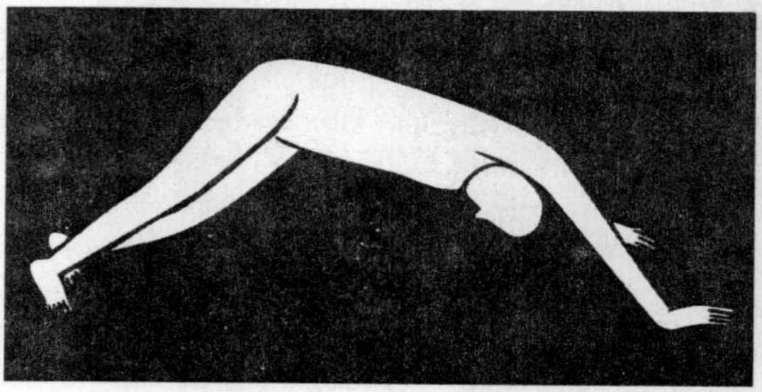

Exercise #5 Step 2.

This can be a difficult posture for those with weak abdomens or low back muscles. Below, you will find a modification of this exercise that I have found useful for those with such conditions. Again, visualize yourself doing the exercise in the most perfect fashion.

STEP 1: Your position is almost the same as in the Step 1 of the unmodified exercise. In this case, your knees rest on the ground.

STEP 2: Bend your knees and allow your behind to move back while your arms straighten and your head drops to the ground.

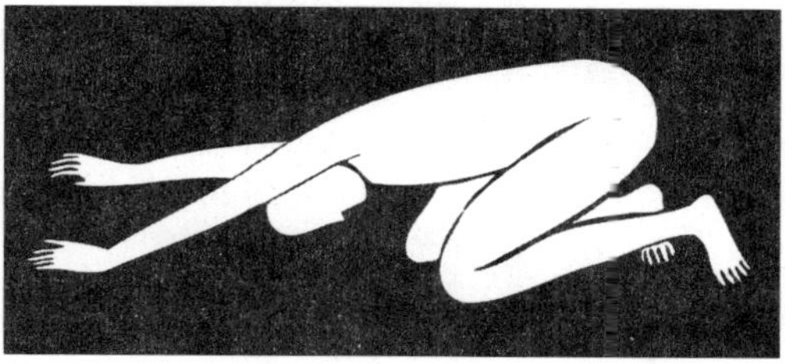

Exercise #5 modified Step 2.

STEP 3: Return to the position of modified Step 1 and repeat.

Over time, experiment to see if your strength has improved enough to do a few of the non-modified or original exercise.

After performing Exercise #5, stand erect with your hands on your hips, breathing in through your nose and out through your mouth a few times. Allow your entire body to relax. (This process was mentioned after doing Exercise #1 and can, in fact, be done following each of the exercises.)

In *Ancient Secrets of the Fountain of Youth*, the British colonel giving the instruction explains that these exercises slow aging and rejuvenate by normalizing the spin of the chakras or psychic vortices in the body:

> "The real benefit of the rites is to normalize the speed of the vortexes. It starts them spinning at a speed which is right for, say, a strong and healthy man or woman 25 years of age.
>
> "In such a person," the Colonel explained, "all the vortexes are spinning at the same rate of speed. On the other hand, if you could see the seven vortexes of the average middle-aged man or woman, you would notice right away that some of them had slowed down greatly. All of them would be spinning at a different rate of speed, and none of them would be working

> together in harmony. The slower ones would be causing nervousness, anxiety, and exhaustion. So, it is the abnormal condition of the vortexes that produces abnormal health, deterioration, and old age."[10]

The colonel's explanation is in keeping with the subtle psychic physiology as described in yogic and tantric texts. Practicing these exercises, however, will be convincing enough in itself.

Rejuvenative Exercise #6

In the medical tantras and literature on advanced meditation practices, there is detailed description of the subtle psychic channels and fluids that permeate the body and maintain health and mental awareness. Of the factors that contribute to aging, the deterioration and loss of function of the channels and dissipation of these subtle substances is crucial. The semen of men and orgasmic fluid of women is said to possess the fluid which, if constantly dissipated, is detrimental to the vitality needed for diligent spiritual practice.

In Hindu and Buddhist tantric practice as well as the Taoist practices of China, retention of this fluid by not allowing for orgasmic release is emphasized. Celibacy is one way to accomplish this. At the same time, all three traditions give methods for inhibiting the urge to ejaculate or release fluid. The Taoist works of Mantak Chia describe such methods and are cited in the Bibliography. These practices are designed to strengthen the genitals and kidneys and allow people to stay relaxed, alert, and in control during intercourse. Ayurvedic books list rejuvenative powders and drinks that can be taken to restore some of the energy dissipated if fluid emission cannot be fully controlled. It should be obvious to the reader that such methods require practice and patience. We in the West are quite inept at understanding the dynamics of sexual energy and how it can be appropriately channeled and utilized. This issue is discussed further in the chapter "Skillful Behavior."

Rejuvenative Exercise #6 is a method of drawing up the vitality of the sexual organs and fluids from the genital region into the entire body. Although Kelder's colonel talks about this exercise in the context of celibacy, Christopher Kilham suggests that it is also an excellent exercise for developing the capability of fluid retention and rechanneling sexual arousal and energy during intercourse. I agree with this and at the same time suggest that people take times for practicing celibacy, using this exercise to help with carnal desire, including the transmutation of sexual frustration, as well as strengthening all of the psychic centers for spiritual purposes or for ordinary life.

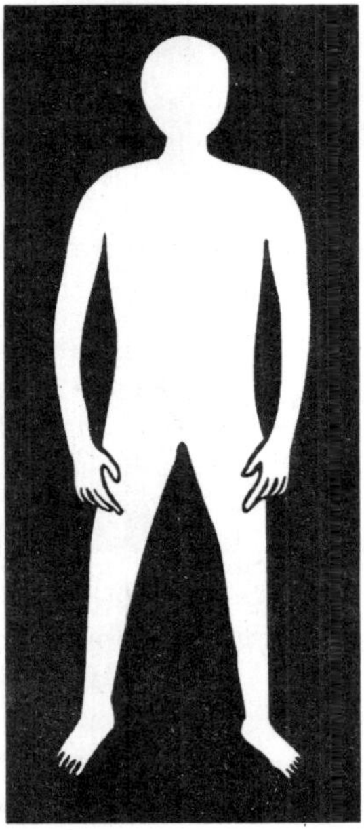

STEP 1: Stand straight with your feet pointing straight forward and your feet shoulder width apart. Rest your tongue on your upper palate. Breathe in.

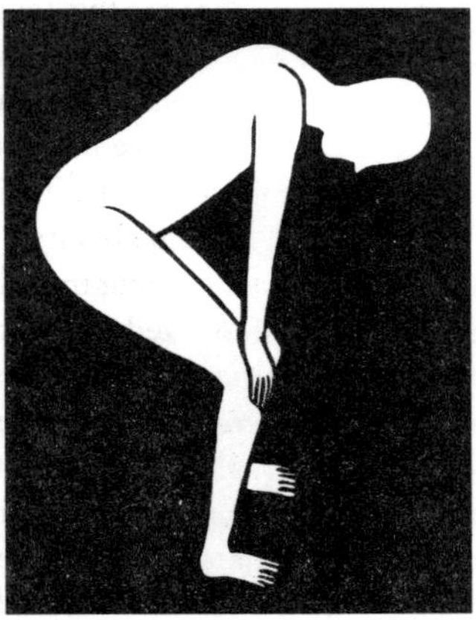

STEP 2: As you exhale bend over from the waist so that your hands rest just above the knees. At this point, all of the air in your lungs is as fully exhaled as possible.

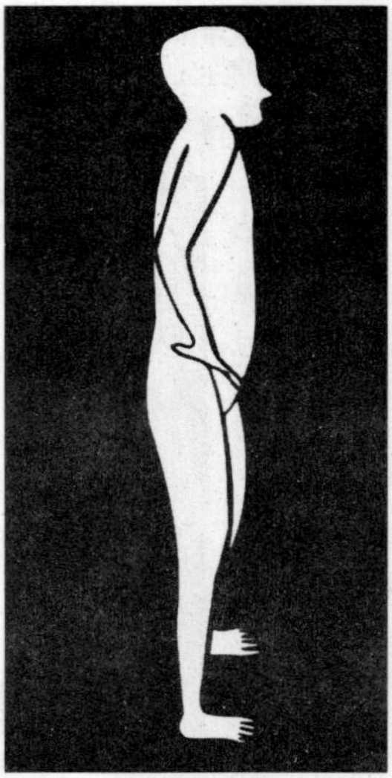

Step 3: Keeping the breath out, straighten yourself up and place your hands on your hips. Press down on your hips and raise your shoulders. At the same time, pull up all of the muscles in your abdomen and groin. If you can feel a pulling up from your genitals, this is even better. Keep looking forward.

When you absolutely have to breathe in, do so and allow your entire body to relax. Breathe in and out a few times so that your breathing rate returns to normal. Then repeat. This exercise need only be repeated three to five times.

In conclusion, Tibetan Rejuvenative Exercises are excellent for all of the seven constitutions. Modifications may be needed, and it may take time to build up to the desired number of repetitions. Be patient with yourself. For such a short and simple series, the physical, psychological, and spiritual benefits of the exercises are great.

YANTRA YOGA

Yantra Yoga is a system of exercise that traditionally was used in retreat situations. As Dr. Rapgay explains, "Yantra Yoga is to help a person to expend as little of his (her) energy to carry out mental and physical activity."[11] In many ways this aim does not differ from the goals of other forms of yoga and martial arts: the utilization of energy in the most efficient way possible by coordinating breath, movement, and concentration. The results are greater efficiency in action, thus promoting longevity and the channeling of energy for more effective spiritual practice. Dr. Rapgay also points out that in solitary retreat, people need to know their body and mind in order to be able to take care of themselves. One key aspect of Yantra Yoga, beyond physical health maintenance and channeling of energy, is that it helps the spiritual adept to remain grounded—to balance the periodic physical abreactions and/or mental flightiness that can arise in spiritual discipline and could possibly be misconstrued as spiritual progress if they were not grounded.

Yantra Yoga is based on the notion of *trul-khor*, or body *(trul)* mandala *(khor)*. The idea here is that the body is the physical manifestation of enlightened potential if we could learn to see and actualize its potentials. Although there are many forms of Yantra Yoga, the core practices are self-massage and five forms of breathing with body postures and movements—all designed to conserve body heat, breathing, and muscle strength. There are approximately seventy-five Yantra Yoga exercises in all.

Because this is a system usually reserved for retreat, the practice of it usually requires a form of initiation. The main proponents of Yantra Yoga practice in the West are Dr. Lobsang Rapgay, who uses the preliminary self-massage aspect in his rejuvenation programs, and the Venerable Namkhai Norbu, Rinpoche. For further information on Yantra Yoga, read *Yantra Yoga* by Namkhai Norbu, Rinpoche (see Bibliography).

RELAXATION THERAPY

The martial arts and yogic traditions of the Orient consider relaxation to be an essential aspect of any exercise or physical healthcare practice. Being in a relaxed state of mind and body when starting exercise will help focus the mind and aid the body in changing into an exercise mode. During exercise, even if the body is working intensely, a relaxed mind ensures that energy is being directed more efficiently. After exercise, relaxation helps the body and mind to integrate the experience of the exercise, thus ensuring greater entrainment and conditioning for future exercise.

Relaxation is not a matter of doing nothing. In the way it is being used here, relaxation is also not the kind of relaxation people experience while sitting back and reading a book or watching television. True therapeutic relaxation does not occur unless there are changes in our brain waves to those frequencies that are indicative of a relaxation response. Unless this occurs, no relaxation is actually ta! :ng place.

In Tibetan medicine and in the medical tantras there is no mention of brain waves. Indeed, it has only been through modern Western technology that measurements of brain activity have been objectively measured. This began with electro-encephalograms used during surgery to measure brain activity, indicating that the person was still alive and had brain function. The range of observable activity from such instrumentation was limited. At times, a patient's brain frequency activity went below this range, a phenomenon for which surgeons had no explanation, and led to emergency procedures in the operating room. Patients, on the other hand, reported experiencing intense but pleasant dreams and visions, being out of their bodies, and having a profound sense of peace. By increasing the frequency ranges of the instrumentation, researchers have been able to observe when and how this happens to the body when such shifts of frequency occur. This is the basis for the modern science of biofeedback.

What is now called the "relaxation response" occurs when brain wave activity is dominated by alpha frequencies. These frequencies are more pronounced during REM sleep and are dominant when measuring the brain activity of people actively engaged in meditation. When alpha brain waves dominate, there is an increase of blood to the brain and a balancing of both central and autonomic nervous system functioning. If people do not get enough alpha brain wave activity in sleep, they will not feel rested, no matter how long they are asleep. Their minds remain discursive, and their bodies stay at a level of alertness that inhibits the replenishment of energy. This can result in many stress-related illnesses. This lack of alpha brain wave stimulation can be caused by single or multiple factors such as poor diet, erratic lifestyle, overstimulation or stimulation deprivation, and emotional and physical crises—all of which can exacerbate each other to create higher levels of stress.

Improvement of diet, lifestyle, and home or general environment help considerably in eliminating stress-related illness. However, learning how to effectively relax—to consciously alter brain wave activity to accentuate alpha—will have the greatest effect. In fact, increasing the dominance of alpha when at rest or active will not only improve physiological functioning but also facilitate better decision making. This will help us in making better choices in diet, lifestyle, and so forth. Thus we can experience more positive effects from the changes we make.

At this point, the distinction should be made between relaxation and meditation, since many Westerners who use relaxation techniques think that they are meditating—and vice versa. Relaxation is a conscious attempt to alter physiology for stress- reduction purposes. Relaxation can also help create the right physical and mental circumstances to go into meditative states of mind. Indeed, meditators are observed to have elevated levels of alpha brain wave activity. But this is a by-product and benefit of the meditative process, not the goal. See the chapter "Meditation and Spiritual Practice" for further discussion of meditation.

Although there are a variety of relaxation techniques, each technique is comprised of fairly similar components: attention to and/or regulation of breathing, an awareness of body sensation which draws our attention inwards, and techniques to stabilize that attention through such procedures as isometrics (a tensing and relaxing of muscles) or guided imagery. Music and sound are also sometimes used. Different people respond to each of the components differently, hence the need for variations in technique. You are advised to try different techniques to find out which one works best for you.

A Three-Part Exercise

The following is a simple Tibetan relaxation exercise as taught by Dr. Lobsang Rapgay. Whereas some relaxation exercises are passive and go very deep, this exercise is more active and is a way of allowing discursiveness of mind to subside and alpha activity to increase during the course of a busy day. It is an excellent exercise in itself but can also be used as a preliminary to meditation.[12]

Part One

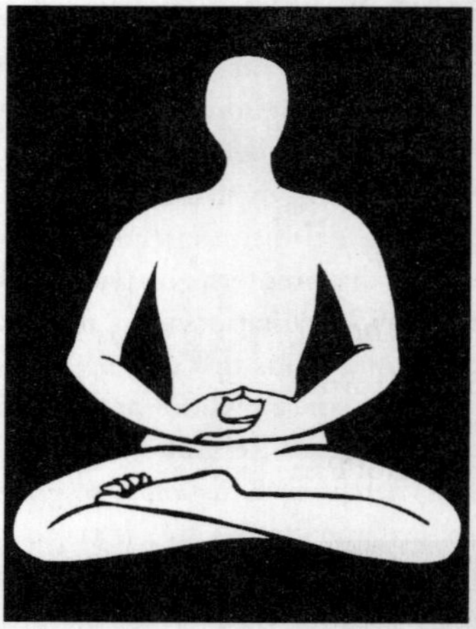

Sit on a cushion with your legs comfortably crossed. To do this, sit on a cushion that is four to six inches high so that your knees are below the level of your navel. This will allow your abdomen to rise and sink without pressure. Rest your hands in your lap. The back of your right hand should rest in the palm of your left hand. Allow your eyes to gently close. Let your tongue rest behind your top front teeth.

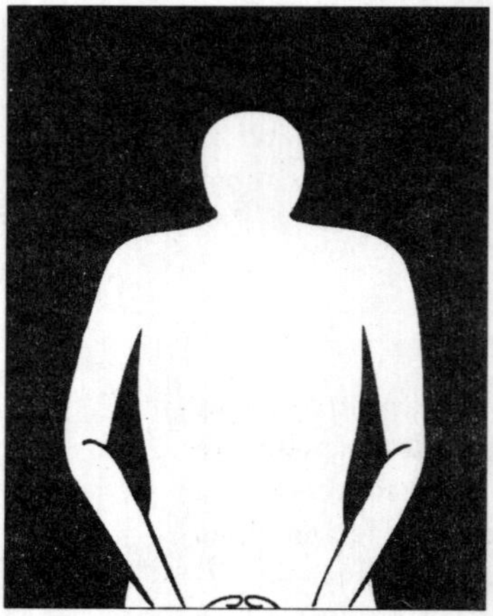

Part Two

STEP 1: While breathing in through the nose to the count of five, raise your shoulders and elbows towards your ears.

STEP 2: Press your right nostril closed with your right middle finger and *breathe out* to the count of five, allowing your shoulders and elbows to settle to their normal position. Repeat this step two more times.

STEP 3: Breath in again as in Step 1, and this time press your left nostril with your left middle finger and breathe out, allowing your shoulders and elbows to come to rest. Repeat this step two more times.

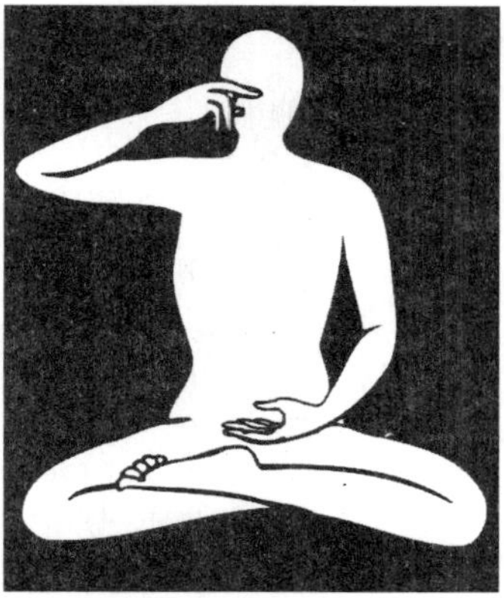

Part Three

STEP 1: *Breathe in* to the count of five, raising both elbows and shoulders as in Step 1 of Part Two.

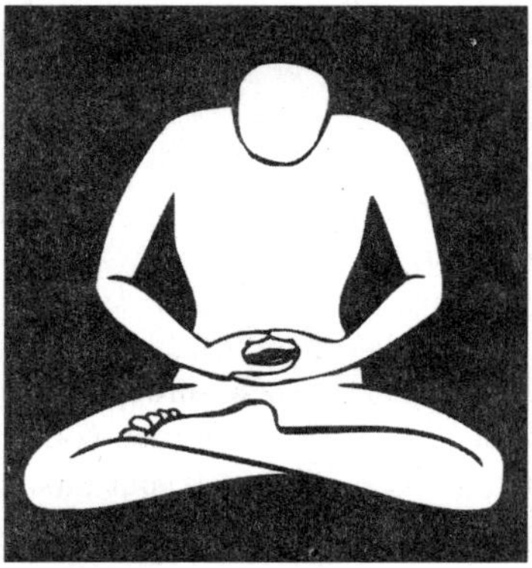

STEP 2: *Breathe out* to the count of five through both of your nostrils; allow your shoulders and elbows to settle and lower your torso slowly, bending at the waist so that your forehead comes as close as possible to the ground in front of you *without* straining.

STEP 3: As you *breathe in* to the count of five, slowly bring your torso to an erect position. *Breathe out* to the count of five.

STEP 4: Remaining upright, *breathe in* to the count of five and *breathe out* to the count of five.

Repeat all steps of Part Three three times in succession.

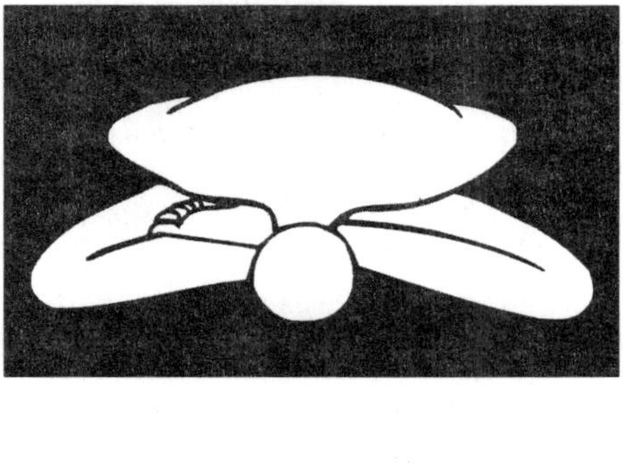

This simple exercise takes five to seven minutes. Most books that deal with relaxation have both short and long exercises. The short ones are designed to slow you down and stabilize your body and mind. The long ones aim at creating a sustained period of alpha brain wave stimulation. Both are encouraged. A short technique such as Dr. Rapgay's is very adaptable and can be practiced at different times during the day. The long forms should be done at times when distraction is at a minimum. When there is time in the day to let go completely and/or make a transition from one activity to the next, the long techniques are most effective. Some people think that such exercises are best if done before bed. Although this will help you sleep better, you will see more benefits on a day-to-day basis if you can train yourself to do such exercises during the day. These relaxation practices are also ideal after any workout program.

The longer forms of relaxation are good for LUNG-types. TrIPA-types should utilize both short and long forms and take advantage of short forms to slow them down. BEKAN-types should use short forms and more active long forms that use isometrics or other more physical means to sharpen their awareness. Imagery with soothing, comfortable, secure scenes are excellent for LUNG-types. Imagery that uses cooling colors and a sense of spaciousness is good for TrIPA-types. BEKAN-types do best if the imagery has brilliant colors and has dynamic, interesting content to prevent them from falling asleep. Any type of music can also be used, provided it conveys the same feeling as the imagery that suits the different constitutions. See the Bibliography for additional resources for learning about relaxation training and biofeedback.

chapter four

SKILLFUL BEHAVIOR

Because of our conditioning and use of language, when most of us hear the words *behavior* or *morality* we think of constraints—constraints which are considered to be primarily from external sources, such as parents, teachers, governments, and so forth. The notion of behaving morally challenges another one of the concepts we hold so dear: freedom.

It is regrettable that we have dichotomized these concepts because the result is to create victims and victors as well as the occasional martyr. Thus, due to our ignorance, attachment, and aggression we choose sides and lose the quality of interconnectedness that exists between freedom and constraint. We reduce our options and our intelligence in handling the world sanely.

Freedom does not mean that we can do anything we want. When we jump, we cannot defy gravity. To get angry at gravity would be senseless and an act of extreme egotism. At the same time, to allow someone or something to have inappropriate control over you without resistance would equally be insane. We need to be able to discriminate, to see situations for what they are.

Teachers, healers, and seers of the past observed what is and is not useful for healthy living and action in the world. By understanding the laws of nature and our true potentials, they were able to develop techniques and rules to help us to maximize those potentials. Some techniques and rules are general and others more specific in that they relate to individual capacities and changing environmental circumstances. Specific techniques and rules are more restrictive for some whose potentials need more refinement, while more lax for those whose capacities allow them to handle greater freedom due to a strong foundation.

The philosophy underlying guidelines for behavior and morality in Tibetan medicine is that all beings want to be happy and free from suffering. This may seem a simplistic statement, but it is actually quite complex. The reason for this is that the Three Poisons distort our perceptions as to what suffering is and what it means to be truly happy. At the same time, on some level we know what works in our life and what doesn't. It is the job of a healer or teacher to provide us with the means to cut through our illusions to gain a clear perception of true and lasting happiness.

The behaviors recommended in Tibetan medicine include behavior towards ourselves and behavior towards others. In this context, morality means that we do not want our behavior to cause suffering to ourselves or others but instead be a means of promoting happiness. If we are not kind and helpful to others and continually put ourselves first, we will inevitably create an inner poverty which will manifest as low self-esteem and doubt. This will in turn be reinforced by a hostile world of our own creation. On the other hand, if we constantly focus on the needs of others, we may overlook the limitations of our resources and fall into a dependent state of being, becoming a burden to others.

Learning how to nurture ourselves and others on the physical, psychological, and spiritual levels demands that we learn what works in the world and how to beneficially handle that knowledge.

Tibetan medicine divides behaviors into categories of general, seasonal, and occasional. The behaviors include dietary considerations (already presented in the chapter "Nutritional Practices"), exercise (see the chapter "Exercise"), sleep, personal hygiene, and interaction with others on physical, emotional, and spiritual levels, including sexual behavior. For Tibetans, sexuality is primarily concerned with how sexual energy and its use can affect overall health and spiritual development.

GENERAL BEHAVIOR — DAILY PRACTICES

In the Ambrosia Heart Tantra, the Buddha, in the form of the Medicine Buddha, gives some basic, sound advice:

> "'Always avoid the two conditions leading to illness (i.e., unwholesome diet and behaviour) by means of mindfulness. Avoid harmful actions of the body, speech, and mind and devote

> yourselves to what is right. Neither torment your senses of taste and so forth nor over-indulge in sensual pleasures.'"[1]

In this way, the Medicine Buddha addresses the Three Poisons. By emphasizing mindfulness, He encourages us to pay attention; to not be so habitual or ignorant. In this way he addresses — BEKAN. By telling us not to torment our senses, He addresses the poison of aggression, thus TRIPA. By drawing our attention towards our tendency to overindulge, He addresses the poison of attachment, associated with LUNG.

In her *Tibetan Buddhist Medicine and Psychiatry*, Terry Clifford is more specific about what is harmful and what the consequences of such actions are:

> Behaviour like sleeping in the day, irregular patterns of eating and sleeping, suppressing natural eliminative instincts and being unaware of the forces of nature and places and how they affect us are further causes of serious disease. Correct actions in the correct environment prevent disease.[2]

The Ambrosia Heart Tantra first addresses situations that are hazardous to life in general such as swimming in large bodies of water, riding wild animals, traveling by night, or traversing steep paths during monsoons. More examples are given with the basic message: know your environment and respect the forces that are there. Some situations cited may be unavoidable or may even be sought out as adventure in our culture. When in reality life is as fragile as a bubble, why should one go out of one's way to risk life and limb? Still, we do. Such situations may make us more mindful. The thrill creates a heightened sense of awareness. However, is this what we need to feel alive? We need to look more closely at our motivations for acting in such ways.

SLEEP

Sleep is important for our body to rest, cleanse, and restore itself. Good sleep is characterized by a preliminary period of rapid eye movement (REM) sleep, an indication of an increase in alpha brain waves, generally dreamless rest, and waking refreshed. If one has many dreams during the night and/or wakes up tired, this is an indication of LUNG imbalance. Beyond traditional recommendations for balancing LUNG, relaxation training during the day is useful in preparation for sleep. And the only dreams worth taking stock of are the ones that occur just before one awakes. It is only these dreams that are considered significant in terms of their symbology and what they portend in an individual's life.

Tibetan medicine encourages people to sleep on their backs or sides rather than on their stomachs. (Sleeping on one's stomach can be an indication of chronic overeating. The exception here are babies, whose digestion is actually helped after they are put on their stomachs to rest.) The yogic way of sleeping is where you lie on your right side, your left knee drawn up with your right hand's fingers positioned accordingly; your little finger sealing the right corner of your mouth; your ring or fourth finger sealing your right nostril; your middle finger on the outside edge of your right eye; and your thumb over your right ear. This is the position of the great reclining Buddha of Thailand and is intended to facilitate cutting through worldly attachment and to enhance spiritual energies in the body. Of all these finger positions, perhaps the most significant and easiest one to practice is the ring finger sealing the right nostril.

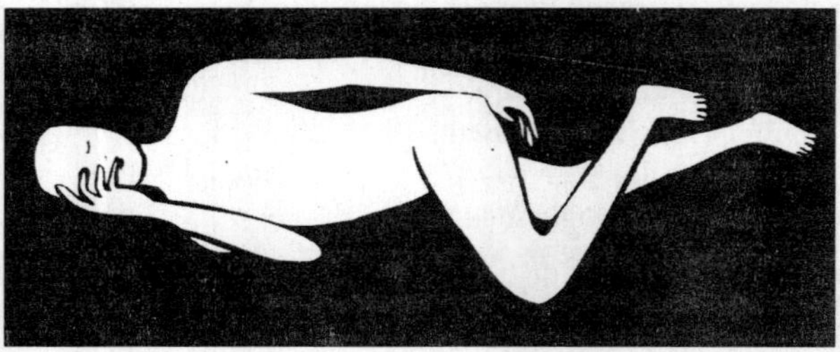

Yogic Sleeping Position.

Try to sleep with your head to the north in the Northern Hemisphere and to the south in the Southern Hemisphere. The point here is to align your body with the earth's magnetic fields. However, if this cannot be done, imagine that your head is lying on the lap of your teacher or some divine being or force that you have confidence in.

Generally, sleeping during the day should be avoided. It aggravates BEKAN and can lead to mental dullness, headaches, sagging skin, and a tendency towards contagious diseases. If one is generally sleeping too much and especially during the day, emetics are encouraged to eliminate excess BEKAN via therapeutic vomiting, and seeking the company of the opposite sex is advised, presumably to raise one's energy. In the early summer where nights are short, a siesta in the afternoon is encouraged. At this time it is also recommended to eat heavy, oily foods in the afternoon. This siesta and dietary recommendation also applies to those who need to rest from an alcoholic hangover, are generally weak, old, or have been traumatized by fear.

If you cannot sleep during the night due to circumstances rather than insomnia, the medical tantras suggest that you do not eat breakfast and try to get the equivalent of half of a normal night's sleep when you can.

Insomnia is a different situation since it does not arise intentionally. People with insomnia are encouraged to drink warm milk, eat heavier foods at night (such as a meat broth), and even drink a small amount of an alcoholic beverage. They are also advised to place a drop of sesame oil on the crown of the head and in the ears before going to bed. If time permits, massaging the bottoms of the feet with sesame oil or taking a warm bath with a couple tablespoons of sesame oil in the water is quite relaxing. There are also Tibetan accupressure series recommended for this condition. In general, you are trying to tame the erratic movement of the internal winds or LUNG.

HYGIENE

Bathing is considered a general health practice. Bathing regularly is said to increase virility, improve complexion and strength, balance body heat, and enhance longevity as well as reduce thirst, itching from accumulated perspiration residues, and lassitude.[3] Please be aware regarding this recommendation that Tibetans rarely had water as hot as we have available for bathing. Nor did they use strong chemicals and detergents on their skin as we do. The above claims are based on scrubbing in tepidly warm or cool water; excessively hot water for bathing is discouraged since it overheats the body and generally depletes energy. Bathing the head with hot water is especially to be avoided since it is injurious to vision and causes hair loss. Those suffering from excessive heat disorders (including fevers), poor digestion, eye complaints, colds, and abdominal bloating or diarrhea should be particularly wary. For such conditions it is also advised not to bathe after eating. The reason for this is that bathing draws circulation to the periphery of the body, drawing heat and blood away from the stomach where it is needed for proper digestion.

As regards soaps, oils, and cosmetics, it is best to use natural, petro-chemical-free products that are in keeping with the nyepa dominance of your constitution. Extensive explanation of the cleansing and health benefits of various cosmetic agents can be found in Melanie Sachs's *Ayurvedic Beauty Care* (see Bibliography). In general, the use of oils rubbed into the skin during self- or administered massage will eliminate tiredness and balance LUNG, thus reducing LUNG symptoms, and slow the aging process. Although not stated in the Ambrosia Heart Tantra, sesame oil is usually what is referred to in this process. However, TrIPA-type constitutions may consider red sandalwood or cold-pressed sunflower oil and BEKAN-types a light amount of a ginger and sesame oil solution. When one is feeling heavy, cold, and generally low in energy, just rubbing oil into the scalp, in the ears, and on the feet can be quite palliative.

Oral hygiene is not mentioned specifically in Tibetan literature. In the diagnosis one is asked to observe the amount of fur, or coating, on the tongue. Such a coating, although varying from constitution to constitution, will be relatively thicker in the morning since it is a digestive waste product. In Indian Ayurveda a silver wire or spoon is used to scrape the tongue of this film. Getting rid of this film will aid digestion.[4] Doing this in addition to rinsing the mouth with warm water will make the mouth feel cleansed. The techniques of brushing and flossing as recommended in the West have their obvious benefits.

SEXUAL INTERCOURSE AND PRACTICES

In recent years, great strides have been made in recognizing the equality of the sexes. This is an important milestone in Western culture—a sign of becoming more civilized. At the same time, most of the changes have occurred in the context of work and responsibility. The only signs of change with regard to sexuality itself have been laws and punishments for crimes of sexual violence to both women and men.

Unfortunately, sexual equality has often come to mean a masculinization of women and a feminization of men. Sexuality and sexual expression remain difficult subjects for us to deal with objectively. This is reflected in the media, where a child can see an extremely violent movie but cannot see a film where two naked people lovingly embrace each other. And, all too often, when sexuality is expressed in the media, it is done in a violent fashion.

Modern psychology has established criteria for what it means to have a "good" relationship — generally a relationship based on truthfulness and mutuality. These ethical and moral principles are no different from those expounded in the Judeo-Christian tradition as well as in Buddhist texts about the sacred bond between beings and, in particular, between men and women. Thus the emotional and spiritual side of relating is well covered. However, in our Western tradition, both secular and sacred, an understanding of the differences between men and women from an energetic point of view is sadly lacking.

In Buddhist literature the ultimate view of men and women is that men represent skillful means and women, wisdom. Without wisdom, skillful means or action in the world becomes out of control and destructive. Without skillful means, wisdom is ineffectual. As beings, we possess both aspects—skillful means and wisdom. It is just that the male body possesses the energy that accentuates skillful means while the female accentuates wisdom. In the process of solitary meditative practice, adepts try to tap into the undeveloped or less dominant aspect (the energy opposite to their gender) in order to bring about a balance of skillful means and wisdom within themselves. This is the meaning of the *yab-yum* found in Buddhist iconography where male and female Buddhas are united in sexual union. These pictures, or *thankas*, should not be taken literally. They represent inner realization and the union of the male and female energies, of skillful means and wisdom, bliss and space. It is enlightenment expressed in its most dynamic from.

At the same time, ordinary sexual embrace is a relative manifestation of this absolute realization, where two people have the opportunity to experience a glimpse of transcendental reality as they lose themselves in union. That is why the dynamics and power of sexuality are considered a sacred matter. In Eastern religion, it is recognized that there are times when, due to blockages in consciousness, a meditator—male or female—might be unable to make shifts to deeper levels of realization. Teachers then advise them to take a consort. The reason for this is that in the circulation of sexual energy there are glimpses of insight and release of blockages. Thus tantric sexual union is also expressed in the literal act of intercourse and other sexual acts. At the same time, the adept is trained to view the sexual act, however enjoyable, not as an end in itself but as a means to an end. It is also a practice where teachers take on students as consorts to help them with their spiritual development.

Such a way of handling sexuality is completely foreign to us—and perhaps not useful to focus on. However, it is necessary to mention this level of sexuality because within spiritual circles and with recognized or self-proclaimed masters it has become a heated subject. This was also true in the East. No doubt, such practices will challenge us to see beyond our conventional perspectives. At the same time, we must be wary of charlatanism and sexual aggrandizement.

For the average person with the usual desires in this material age, the morality around sex as expounded in the tantras is useful to follow. Desire that leads to attachment aggravates LUNG. Thus the texts talk about not dwelling on or indulging oneself constantly with what is beautiful and sensually pleasing. Some may think that if we indulge the senses we would pacify desire, but in fact the opposite occurs. The more we satisfy such heightened desire, the more the pattern of seeking what is desired is strengthened. This is the basis of addiction, and I have heard many recovering addicts say that they were convinced that if they had just one more drink, one more snort, that would be enough.

As regards appropriate and inappropriate partners, the thirteenth chapter of the second book of the *Gyud-Zhi* says, "One should not indulge in intercourse with animals, nor with wicked or dishonourable persons, pregnant women, weak women or women during menstruation."[5] The reasons for these restrictions vary. Presumably one does not have sex with animals due to the potential for disease but also the harm one does to the animal. It is basically a violation of morality in that it is not a natural act for either the animal or the person and is not, therefore, an act of mutuality. It is taking advantage of another being. On a subtler level, the psychic and subtle energies of a human are not the same as those of an animal; thus in the movement of energy during a sexual act, imbalance of bodily forces leading to further suffering is likely inevitable.

By "dishonourable people" the Ambrosia Heart Tantra alludes to adultery and having sexual relations with people you dislike (because of exploitation, revenge, boredom, and so forth). Although it sounds moralistic, this advice is given from the highest tantric level of awareness. The body is basically the residing place of all elements, which, from the absolute point of view are manifestations of divine forces. Our bodies are comprised of subtle channels and essences that once mixed and entwined with another person, leave lasting impressions on us. Do not most "liberated" Westerners and others recall their first sexual encounter? Feelings, memories, even body sensations, the psycho-physical residues of such intimate contact, persist. Such sensations can often present blockages to establishing similar or deeper contact with a spouse or more permanent partner. Neuroses, guilt, feelings of inadequacy, unrealistic expectations, and wanderlust all can result. In cultures that are not homogeneous with varying or loose social rules, the emotional consequences of such actions coupled with the subtle energy memories may be the cause of lack of intimacy and ability to commit to a relationship.

The reasons for advice not to engage in intercourse with pregnant, weak, or menstruating women are physiological. Although in many cultures and even in Tibetan culture, intercourse during pregnancy is sometimes allowed, the general recommendation is to abstain. Deep penetration is to be avoided, especially towards the end of pregnancy where it can create great discomfort for the woman. And although there are differing opinions about ejaculation within a woman at this time, the Venerable Kalu Rinpoche, a highly revered Tibetan yogi, states that the seminal fluid creates the experience of burning for the baby and that the insertion of a penis into the vagina during pregnancy makes the baby feel that it is being beaten with a hot poker.

As regards "weak" women, the medical texts teach that intercourse and/or sexual excitement may weaken a woman further, aggravating the balance of the LUNG nyepa. As the text does not specify what is meant by "weak," the recommendation should be considered general. A further point on this matter is that the considerations made here may have to do with the Buddhist sense of mutuality in interaction. How much is a man considering how a woman feels in these circumstances? However, in both Taoism and Hindu tantra, it is said that sex can at times be therapeutic. In the context of illness, Terry Clifford talks about the therapeutic effects of intercourse in mental illness,[6] but other illnesses are not specified. For greater clarification readers are encouraged to study the books on Taoist sexual practices cited in the Bibliography.

In both Taoism and Hindu tantra, the retention of sexual fluids is a practice designed to strengthen the body and transmute these substances for higher spiritual purposes. These same practices exist in Tibetan medical tradition, but they are not considered relevant to the average person. Hindu tantra and Taoist teaching insist that such practices be done with a spiritual emphasis and in a disciplined fashion, but it seems that such practices were considered more commonplace than in the Tibetan context, where they were primarily the domain of the Tibetan yogic way of life.

In spiritual practice, the yogi works with the male and female energies of the body, particularly aspects of the subtle energy body called the winds, channels, and drops. Too esoteric to explain here, the point is to raise and strengthen the sexual force in the body which will be experienced at the tip of the penis or clitoris of the respective male or female. The retention of seminal fluids and sexual force does not come about through brute force or neurotic repression. It is a subtle matter demanding an understanding of the subtle energy physiology and a level of realization of the Buddhist principle of emptiness. The passion of ordinary beings is being transformed into the compassion of the yogi. Thus such practices require spiritual training and moral commitment. For the average person, although positive motivation and compassion may be present in the act of making love, the loss of seminal fluids will result in the loss of this subtle energy and a more rapid depletion of overall body energy and vitality. The medical tantras make recommendations to minimize the effects of the loss to the body of such seminal fluids. The emphasis is on semen since men are more prone to larger losses and the resultant harmful effects. In this matter, women are considered superior. A woman's fluid release takes longer, and the supply is greater; still, women can also squander this resource.

During the winter, as the body tries to maintain its warmth, BEKAN is more present or accentuated in our constitution. The result is that sperm and seminal fluid is more abundant, and it is said, therefore, that intercourse can occur without restriction in frequency. In the fall, intercourse is permissible every other day. In the summer and monsoon season (presumably also springtime), intercourse with the release of fluid should happen no more than once every two weeks. If engaged in more frequently, the result will be the dulling of the senses, possible dizziness, and a shortened life.

Such restrictions may seem rather strict, but they are designed to enhance life, prolong the body's vital force, and allow for spiritual progress. At the same time, there are virilification practices and substances mentioned in the texts to help those who indulge too much in sexual activity or have problems of impotence or infertility. Some are included in the chapter "Detoxification and Rejuvenation." Other methods can be found in sources for Tibetan medicine cited in the Bibliography.

Other Sexual Practices

In the *Tibetan Arts of Love*, Gedun Chopel discusses other forms of experiencing sexual pleasure. Along with classical foreplay, postures for intercourse are elucidated as are practices of oral sexual gratification.

In the precepts taken by a lay Buddhist practitioner, mention is made of inappropriate sexual acts. Inappropriate partners have already been discussed. However, some teachers also classify oral sex, masturbation, and homosexual sex as inappropriate. Without delving into the details concerning each, the reasoning for such admonitions is that such acts often create extreme desire, the result being the imbalance of LUNG. Of the three, I have only found reference to oral sex in the literature. Gedun Chopel includes it as part of caressing and the playful aspect of erotic pleasure.[7] Again, mutuality and respect for a partner are emphasized. He does not go as far as in the Hindu tradition where one views the partner as divine and drinks the vaginal or penile secretions as nectar.[8] However, as in Tibetan tradition, to be base and lustful in such an act is a violation of one's partner and only creates heightened levels of neurotic preoccupation and attachment. While such ideas are not expressed in any of the medical or Buddhist tantras thus far examined, approaching such sexual practices from a more enlightened and mutual perspective is advised if such practices are to be indulged in. Regarding the moral or religious implications of such acts, in reference to oral sex the Venerable Kalu Rinpoche has said:

> There is some basis for this prohibition in the teachings of the dharma. However, it seems to me that these are relatively minor points which we could let alone, and just let sentient

> beings in samsara be sentient beings in samsara. I am not going to be too particular about the whole thing.[9]

SPIRITUAL PRACTICES — CULTIVATING TRUE HEALTHINESS

As explained in the chapter "Self Evaluation" and in Appendix One, the constitution we currently have is the direct result of our previous actions—our past karma. It is the reference point from which we experience our world and interact either harmoniously or unharmoniously with body, speech, and mind. It is our blueprint for enlightenment.

This being the case, life finds its highest expression in spiritual endeavors and when we act in the world from whatever degree of spiritual realization we have thus far attained. All of the recommendations made in the medical tantras are designed to facilitate spiritual growth and progress. Thus it is only logical and natural that there are general spiritual practices on the levels of body, emotions, and spirit included in the recommendations for daily behavior.

Dr. Yeshe Donden succinctly sums up these recommendations given by the tantras:

> *Physically*, even if now we are not Bodhisattvas and are not capable of giving our own bodies to others, we can give gifts to others; we can give blood to others who do not have enough. Persons who make organ donations are indeed carrying out the Bodhisattva precepts. *Verbally*, we should use our speech with an attitude of altruism; for instance, if another is seeking to kill someone and trying to find out where they are, even if you had seen the victim, you can tell the killer that you do not know where that person is and thereby free that being from being killed (and free the killer from the karma of physically killing someone—the author). Similarly, *mentally* you should think about what will be helpful to others, discriminating between what helps and what harms others.[10]

The ethical and moral considerations voiced here are similar to those found in other world traditions. One should not kill, steal, lie, and so forth. Besides acts that we may personally commit, the tantras also speak of how to interact with people to create upliftment as well as situations that should be avoided in order to prevent negative consequences for ourselves and others. Such rules are not divine edicts, but formulations from the clear insight of beings with an awakened state of mind, the purpose of which is to help ourselves and others and to avoid suffering now and in the future.

When perpetrating a negative act against another person, the suffering we experience will be one of moral and spiritual poverty. As we commit such acts, we lose our self-esteem. Our lifestyle begins to show signs of deterioration. We then begin to suffer in more obvious ways—mentally and physically. The classic Buddhist text on the results of negative actions is Dharmaraksita's *The Wheel of Sharp Weapons:*

> When no matter how well-meant our actions towards others,
> They always elicit a hostile response,
> This is the wheel of sharp weapons returning
> Full circle upon us for wrongs we have done.
> Till now we have repaid loving-kindness with malice;
> Hereafter let's always accept others' favours
> Both graciously and with most humble respect.[11]

The tantras are explicit in demonstrating the causal relationship between our intentions and the actions we engage in vis-a-vis our world and our physical, emotional, and spiritual well-being. It is only because of our materialistic perspective that such insights into the effects of our actions seem parochial.

True healthiness is expressed in our actions of body, speech, and mind towards ourselves and others. With respect to ourselves we can create a lifestyle that sustains life and a view of ourselves that promotes a sense of self-esteem. As we are kinder and gentler to ourselves, we can naturally extend these qualities to others. The deeper meaning of this is a recognition of our true potential and the desire to create the circumstances in which they can manifest. This is the greatest gift we can give to ourselves.

Giving others the teaching, guidance, and support to

experience the same is the greatest act of altruism. Natural, spontaneous, and joyful willingness to act in such a way towards others is the highest testimony of a truly healthy person. Seeing the world as an interdependent whole, it is only logical that the ethical application of what is useful to promote our own well-being is extended to others. It is not a question of going to some distant place called hell if we do not act in such a way, but rather that if we do not act in such a way, we and others experience hell in our suffering here and now. This is not given as a warning or admonition but as a simple fact of life. Specific meditations and spiritual information is provided in the following chapter.

SEASONAL BEHAVIOR

The topic of seasonal behavior in the medical tantras deals with what behaviors we should be mindful of in different climates and during seasonal changes.

From one season to the next our environment places different demands on our bodies. In cold weather our bodies try to generate heat to secure proper body function. In hot weather our body cools down. In dry weather our body tries to maintain the physiological mechanisms for moisturization.

Each change of temperature, barometric pressure, and moisture level stimulates or challenges different organ systems and tissues of our bodies. This is also true for our psychological dispositions. For example, it is recognized that the amount of sunlight a person experiences can affect mood. For the most part we are incapable of manipulating such circumstances unless, of course, we take a vacation, move, and so forth. What we can all do, however, is to make changes in our diets, exercise, and our habits to help our bodies adjust to environmental circumstances more efficiently. We need to be flexible in order to adapt. This month's healthy diet may be the cause of next month's aches and pains. An exercise we do vigorously at one time may need to be done more gently or not at all at other times.

One of the primary foci of the tantra's material for seasonal behavior changes has to do with the alteration of dietary practices, the emphasis being on the tastes and qualities of the food that best work with the energetics of the given season, within the context of one's particular constitution. Each constitution is benefited by three tastes as indicated in the chapter "Nutritional Practices." Thus when making food choices, *try to accentuate the taste that reflects both your constitution and the seasonal energetics.* Beyond diet, exercise, and hygiene, specific cleansing or detoxification procedures such as enemas, purgatives, and emetics are given. See the chapter "Detoxification and Rejuvenation" for a more detailed explanation.

Winter Solstice to Early Spring

(Northern Hemisphere: December 21 to February 3)
(Southern Hemisphere: June 21 to August 3)

Generally this is the coldest and darkest time of the year. Plant life dies back from the surface of the ground and recedes into the roots to build up energy for the spring. Animals hibernate or slow down their activity. Such action is done to store and conserve energy.

To prevent the dissipation of energy due to cold, dress warmly (especially around the waist, the back, and the ears, areas which relate to the kidneys and water element energy of the body) and stay in warm environs. Do not exercise to the point of perspiration since the dissipation of heat from the body will be difficult to replace. Bathing should be done less frequently for the same reason. To help close the pores rub the body with sesame oil after bathing.

This is not a time to eat raw fruits, juices, salads, and so forth. Nor is it a time to fast. It is a time to stoke the fires, eating warming cooked stews, soups, and so forth. If you eat meat, it is better to increase the amount at this time. Also, oiliness in the diet can be increased. The tastes of food should be primarily sour, salty, and sweet. People of LUNG constitutions should be particularly mindful in following these recommendations.

Early Spring through Equinox to Late Spring

(Northern Hemisphere: February 4 to early May)
(Southern Hemisphere: August 4 to early November)

Because of the slowness of activity and the richness of the diet needed during the winter, the sticky, thick quality of BEKAN arises as a natural by-product. If this quality is not eliminated in a natural, healthy manner, the result can be early spring colds, flus, and other forms of lymphatic congestion. The major factors contributing to this situation are that as the spring sun brings more warmth and light, the body no longer needs to maintain the same level of metabolic heat, especially digestive heat. As digestive heat cools down, the ability to absorb the rich diet and the specified tastes of winter decreases.

At this time of year the diet should be lighter and the tastes emphasized bitter (such as found in herbs and spring greens), hot (spiced), and astringent (astringent foods are those that do not fit into any other taste category). If meat is consumed, it should be from animals that come from a dry climate (e.g., buffalo or bison). To break down the accumulation of BEKAN, drink ginger tea with honey.

Exercise is encouraged during this time as a way of stimulating lymphatic elimination. Get out into the air and breathe pleasant fragrances. The use of a mini-trampoline or inversion apparatus to hasten lymphatic cleansing is useful. Hygiene should emphasize the cleansing of excessive oiliness accumulated from the previous season. Bringing up a sweat through vigorous walking or running followed by rubbing the body with red lentil flour is recommended.[12] To eliminate excess BEKAN in the form of sinus or stomach mucus, emetics to induce vomiting may be needed. Because the body is getting rid of the oily, weighty quality of winter, there can be a stale smell to the body. The Ambrosia Heart Tantra suggests sitting in pleasant-smelling gardens for one's own (but possibly also others') benefit. Dr. Donden is more direct in suggesting the use of fragrances and perfumes. Because such substances can either block the skin and create negative reactions or enhance body beauty and health, quality and constitutionally appropriate products should be emphasized. People of BEKAN-type constitutions should be particularly mindful of these recommendations. Refer to Melanie Sachs's *Ayurvedic Beauty Care* listed in the Bibliography.

Early Summer

(Northern Hemisphere: early May to early August)
(Southern Hemisphere: early November to early February)

In the West we tend to think this is the greatest time to be outdoors. We jog at noon, sunbathe, or work up a sweat in the garden. We overheat our bodies and then try to cool them down in air-conditioned rooms and swimming pools, or with ice-cold drinks. Although it is necessary to cool the body down at this time, the extremes we go to are a response to overheating our bodies at this time. We overdo and thus overcompensate, resulting in greater weakness and susceptibility to illness in subsequent seasons. Some symptoms of overheating may be skin rashes, blistering, migraines, or diarrhea. Such bodily reactions may necessitate the use of an herbal or oil purgative.

Generally, it is recommended to avoid staying in the sun for prolonged periods, especially during the hottest times of the day. Exercise should emphasize relaxation rather than exertion. Try to conduct your activities as much as possible in the shade, especially eating. Rather than crank up the air conditioner, wear light clothing made of cotton or other fibers that allow the body to breathe. The emphasis on hygiene should be on cooling, relaxing baths without chilling the body. The use of fragrances is encouraged to deal with increased perspiration and the fact that foods putrify more easily at this time. The diet should not be heavy at this time but emphasize the taste of sweet and the qualities of light, slightly oily, and cooling. This is the time for more fruits and salads as well as cool water and beverages. Alcohol, if taken, should be diluted with water. Hot (spicy), salty, and sour foods should be avoided since they contribute to body heat. As the heat of the environment is intensified we should be taking compensatory measures to allow the body to stay cool. This is especially true for the TRIPA-types.

Late Summer through Early Winter

(Northern Hemisphere: early August to mid-December [solstice])
(Southern Hemisphere: early February to mid-June [solstice])

In the classic literature, the season we call autumn is referred to as the monsoon season. It is generally a time when there is increased rain and moisture and a gradual cooling of the winds. This is also considered a variable time, where temperatures vacillate more. The added moisture can increase problems with BEKAN-types while the winds and variability challenge LUNG-types.

It is necessary to be prepared for sudden changes in weather; for example when wearing light clothing, carry a jacket, raincoat, or umbrella. Bathing should be in tepid to warm water since the warmth is a way of ensuring greater immune resistance.

With regard to diet, this is the time of greatest harvest. Most of the foods of this time require cooking to be broken down enough for the body to metabolize them. The tastes to focus on are sour, salty, and sweet—in that order. Sweet foods, which normally have a cooling effect, should be eaten warm, such as cooked fruit sauces, purées, and pies. Food should also be a little heavier and oilier than in summer. By keeping foods warm, but not too heavy, one is discouraging metabolic body heat loss. This helps the body to start building up its heat reserves for the impending winter.

This is a time when the use of enemas may be needed to deal with digestive sensitivity. Other symptoms that may be noted are allergies, gas, constipation, and tension headaches. Following the seasonal recommendations provided will help to abate these conditions and prepare one for winter.

OCCASIONAL BEHAVIOR

The primary emphasis in the tantras' presentation of occasional behavior is purification and allowing the body to function without repressing natural urges.

What is meant by natural urges are the means by which the body nutrifies itself and eliminates. Sometimes out of habit, social convention, or sheer ignorance we don't eat or drink when thirsty, try to avoid sleep, or block the release of a sneeze, belch, or intestinal gas. In all such cases, the LUNG energy of the body is disturbed. Since LUNG is involved with the experience of sensation in various regions of the body as well as the movement of airs and liquids, denying these sensations or not releasing substances will cause derangement of the nyepas; this results in more pains and distress in the body later on. Not knowing how suppression of body urges can cause such symptoms we may seek medical advice and undergo unnecessary treatments when we need only to cease the suppression and follow the simple remedies provided in the tantras.

The fifteenth chapter of the *Gyud-Zhi* gives the consequences of suppressing natural tendencies and some useful remedies to overcome the resulting problems. For the sake of simplification, a chart of urge, symptom of suppression, and remedy is provided. Some of the remedies can be readily applied while others require knowing formulas for medicinal baths and herbal solutions. For these you are advised to contact a Tibetan Ayurvedic practitioner.

IF YOU SUPPRESS THE URGE TO . . .	THE SYMPTOMS THAT ARISE MAY BE . . .	THE REMEDIES ARE . . .
eat	disturbed appetite, body weakness, localized abdominal pain, dizziness	A snack of light, warm slightly oily foods (meat or noodle broth). Avoid over-eating to compensate
drink	dry mouth, dizziness, forgetfulness, loss of clarity, heart problems	cool foods, perhaps some fruit. Avoid excessively cold or hot drinks
hiccup	senses weakened, headaches, stiffness in limbs, distorted cheeks	Look at the sun. Inhale smoke of aloewood and sandalwood nasally
yawn	senses weakened,headaches stiffness in limbs, distorted cheeks	foods and medicines to pacify LUNG conditions

IF YOU SUPPRESS THE **URGE** TO . . .	THE **SYMPTOMS** THAT ARISE MAY BE . . .	THE **REMEDIES** ARE . . .
sneeze	dampened senses, one-side neck pain, headaches, loss of strength in cheeks	Look at the sun. Inhale smoke of aloewood and sandelwood nasally to clear sinus passages
saliva/spit	dizziness, nasal drip, weight and appetite loss heart ailments, breathing and swallowing difficulties	alcoholic beverages. rest, pleasant conversation
throat mucus/spit	more mucus accumulation, hiccups, weight and appetite loss, breathing and swallowing difficulties, heart ailments	warm drink made of raw sugar, piper long pepper (pippli), and ginger boiled together (suggested ratio: 3x sugar, 1x pepper, and 1x ginger)
breathe	dulling of mental clarity, tumor formation, heart disease	rest, warming foods (especially after exercise or fatigue) (LUNG pacifying)
vomit	breathing difficulties, loss of appetite, skin disease (both acute and chronic) itching eyes, leprosy, lower body swelling, contagious diseases	fasting, inhaling the smoke of aloewood and sandalwood, washing the mouth with the same woods, purgatives
sleep	yawning, heaviness in head, weakened digestion and eyesight	massage, rest, eat light warm, slightly fatty foods
cry	pain in the eyes, dizziness, catarrh, loss of appetite, pain in head and heart	sleep, cheerful company, alcoholic beverages
pass/intestinal gas	poor digestive heat, heart ailments, dry stool, constipation, weak eyesight, abdominal pain, tumors	abdominal oil massage and/or herbal enemas, fermented foods (i.e., sauerkraut miso) to activate gas elimination

IF YOU SUPPRESS THE **URGE** TO . . .	THE **SYMPTOMS** THAT ARISE MAY BE . . .	THE **REMEDIES** ARE . . .
have bowel movement	cramps, colds, pain in brain, colic, impaired vision, tumors, disturbed digestion, heart disease, fecal backup, vomiting	sesame oil massage, herbal enemas, soak in medicinal waters, bathing, taking herbal medicines
urinate	abdominal pain, kidney stones, tumors, weak eyesight, heart and bladder disease, disturbed digestion, reproductive organ disease	oil massage, oil enemas, medicines taken through penis or vaginally, supplementation (herbs)
ejaculation or sexual substance release	penile diseases, impotence, fever, throbbing in heart, testicular swelling, pain in limbs, difficulty with urination, disturbed eyesight and other senses	include sesame oil, chicken and meat, milk, millet in diet medicinal baths, relaxing, alcoholic beverages, have intercourse

As mentioned in the section on "Occasional Behavior," the tantras discuss the importance of proper elimination and purification. The Ambrosia Heart Tantra says, "Good purification makes for a complete cure and an absence of ailments."[13]

Purification in the bodily sense is an important aspect of the therapy known as *Len Nga* (Sanskrit—*Pancha Karma*). Len Nga, or Pancha Karma, means "five actions." These actions are intended to cleanse, renutrify, and rejuvenate the body. There are different ways in which the body is purified, and each one of these ways is best done in accordance with a person's constitution and presenting conditions. Elaboration of these methods and when they are most appropriate is found in the chapter "Detoxification and Rejuvenation."

chapter five

MEDITATION AND SPIRITUAL PRACTICE

Any holistic approach to health involves taking responsibility for one's life. To be responsible does not imply being burdened with something. Rather, responsibility means the ability to respond. In order to respond to a situation most effectively, we need to develop a clear sense of what the situation is. How well do we understand our environment, the demands being placed on us by time and considerations? Do we have a clear grasp of what our potentials are and how best to use them?

More often than not, the reason why what we do in the world does not work is due to the fact that we misperceive situations, have preconceived ideas about how we want things to work out, and then negotiate or, if need be, do battle with those around us to get our way. Such behavior is a result of the Three Poisons of ignorance, attachment, and aggression.

In our discussions of constitutions and the various means available in Tibetan Ayurveda and healing arts to return us to the optimal functioning of our nyepa, importance has been placed on utilizing our abilities to deepen our spiritual lives, to create a source of lasting joy for ourselves and others. True health is indicated by how we demonstrate a loving care for ourselves and others. It is an active demonstration that we are cutting through ignorance, attachment, and aggression to a more awakened state of being.

Such a state of being does not usually happen overnight. It should be obvious from the material presented that one needs to develop skills of contemplation and self-reflection in order to see the world more clearly and act more effectively. To change diet, exercise appropriately, and deal with changes of behavior based on circumstances, one needs to develop a flexible, open mind. Without this flexibility, such changes will be dogmatic in nature, the result being some form of fanaticism which one inflicts on oneself and possibly others. Meditation is a means of preventing this by creating flexibility and openness.

An old Zen saying is, "Do not look for the truth. Only cease to cherish opinions." Opinions, no matter how accurate, are founded on preconceptions. Meditation is about cutting through preconceptions. It is concerned with opening ourselves up beyond what our ego narrowly defines us as being while not becoming morosely self-absorbed or self-conscious. Meditation is about allowing that which is natural and wholesome within us to function as a source for creative action in the world. Implicit in this approach is the premise that we are basically good and that our true nature is in touch with reality. Given the opportunity to express ourselves without being blinded by ignorance, attachment, and aggression, our actions are spontaneous and correct, with regard to ourselves and others. Since the Three Poisons are also the basis of the nyepas, through meditative practice we are, in fact, beginning to address the causal factors in our experience of separateness from the world. We thus address our original blueprint, or self-created map, and begin to wind our way through the labyrinth of our lives towards a reunification with our world. We become stronger physically, emotionally, and spiritually.

Because of our different constitutions, we each have different issues that arise through the process of meditation. Depending on the issues facing individuals in their spiritual evolution and the types of people they are, meditations need to be varied. Some people need to focus on attachment or ignorance. Other people need to have meditations that are silent while some need music or visual stimulation. The medical tantras themselves do not specify types of meditation. However, in the past doctors were more frequently priests or monks and would rely on their religious backgrounds to find meditative processes best suited to the individuals whose healings they were directing.

The meditations presented in this book are of a generic type that can be used by all people, regardless of religious persuasion or constitutional mix. All world traditions have prayers and meditative practices. Although you may find that the techniques and guidelines presented here are useful and complete in themselves, they can also be used as a foundation from which to deepen your own prayer and meditative life.

WHAT IS MEDITATION?

Meditation is not the same as relaxation. Relaxation is an attempt to create a specific physiological and psychological effect through altering brain wave patterns. In meditation, brain wave patterns are altered, but this is a by-product. Meditation is a process where you learn to be present in whatever state you happen to be in. This "being present" is the foundation for deeper exploration.

Meditation is not intended to make the mind go blank. A void mind is a scary notion for some people and is often the reason used by religious zealots for instilling fear in people to not do meditation. ("An empty mind is the devil's playground.") The truth is that *you cannot void your mind.* There are approximately 60,000 mind moments in every second of thought. Due to our habit patterns, we screen out and identify with certain impressions which in turn give our thought process the illusion of continuity and solidity. This is a self-limiting process. Meditation is an attempt to free up our fixation on one impression over another. The result is greater relaxation, more fluidity in seeing things with new freshness, and a greater sense of possibility.

Meditation is not hypnosis. Truthfully speaking, unless we are conscious and awake, we are living our lives in a hypnotic state, believing in and following illusions, without giving much thought as to how they arise. Meditation is intended to be an active process where one maintains focus on whatever the subject of the meditation is. In our everyday lives, this attentiveness helps us to dispel illusions and see things for what they are, rather than being carried away in a phantasm of our own creation.

Some meditative processes involve visualization. Visualization is not the same as imagery. Imagery is an illusion designed to affirm or direct psycho-physical processes for the purpose of creating a certain state of being based on preconceived notions. In the truest sense, visualization is the process of trying to unmask reality and see it for what it is by utilizing the vision of reality as experienced by those whose seeing is undistorted.

MEDITATION ON EQUANIMITY

The purpose of this meditation technique is to allow for the establishment of equanimity—a calm and clear mind.

Our minds are like agitated pools of water filled with mud and silt. We may know that the water is basically clean and fresh, but we are at a loss to figure out how to get the mud and silt out of it because of the agitation. We could try to extract the mud and silt gradually, but this can be time consuming and waste much effort. On the other hand, we could try to calm the agitation in the water, so the mud and silt settle and we are left with the clean and fresh water. We can then taste the water and appreciate it for what it is. In the same way, developing calmness in our minds brings us in touch with a wholesomeness about who we are. Like tasting the water for the first time, we develop a deeper sense of appreciation in our aliveness. And like the clarity of a still pool, we begin to see things clearly, without distortion.

The meditation technique we use here has existed for thousands of years and is used in a variety of religious and secular settings. It is very simple and as with most things that are simple, quite profound. One should try to establish a regular routine of practice (a quiet place, a special time) and allow for at least twenty minutes.

The main emphasis in this technique is on the breath. However, unlike breathing exercises where you are trying to breath a certain way, this technique relies on a passive observation of the natural movement of breathing—in and out. Thus you are focusing on what keeps you alive from moment to moment.

Steps to the Meditation

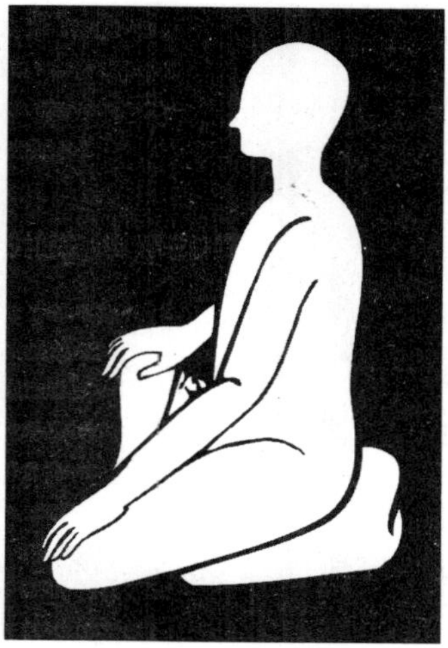

STEP 1: Get yourself into a comfortable sitting position. If you are on a chair, sit as upright as you can, slightly away from the back of the chair if possible, your feet resting firmly on the ground. Rest your hands on the tops of your thighs, palms down. If you are sitting on the ground, place yourself on a semi-firm or firm cushion that is at least four to six inches thick. Cross your legs in a manner that allows your knees to be lower than your navel. Allow your spine to be straight, yet comfortable. Let your hands be palms down and resting at or just above your knees.

STEP 2: Your head should be positioned so that your chin is slightly tucked, your tongue resting behind your top front teeth, with your lips loosely together or just slightly parted. Your eyes should be slightly open with your gaze towards the ground down the line of your nose. If sitting on a chair, gaze between your knees toward the ground; if sitting on the ground, gaze approximately eighteen inches from the point at which your legs are crossed.

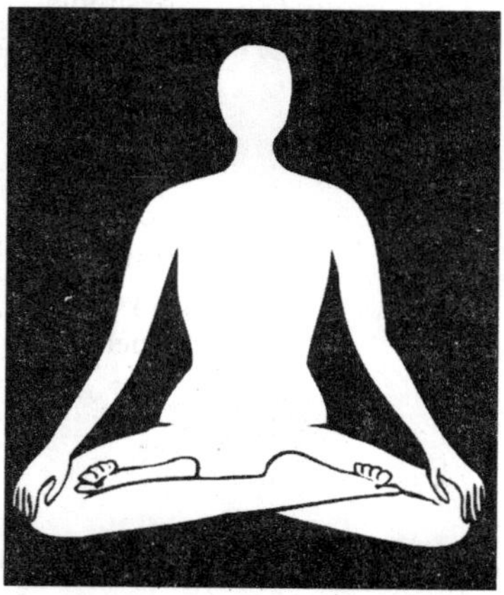

Lotus meditation pose.

STEP 3: Breathe in through your nostrils slowly and then tense your abdomen, groin, and behind. Hold your breath for a moment and then release the tension and your breath so that you allow yourself to settle in a relaxed way onto the cushion that you rest on. Become aware of allowing your diaphragm to soften so that your belly rises and sinks naturally with each breath.

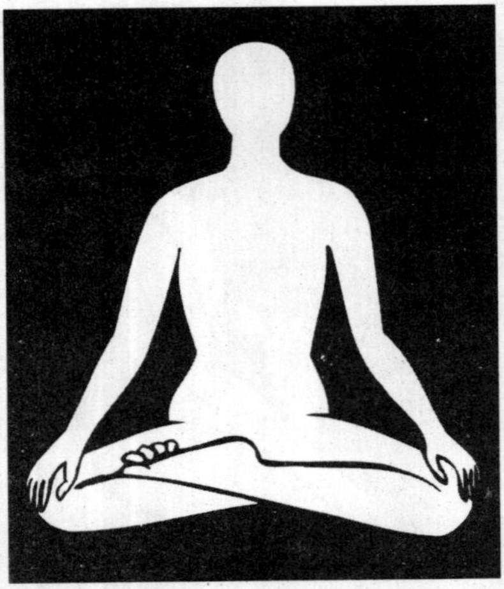

STEP 4: Now focus your attention on your breathing at the tip of your nostrils. As the air comes in, you are aware that it allows your abdomen to expand. As you breathe out, become aware of the sensation of air moving at the tip of your nostrils. Focus particularly on this sensation and get a sense that the air moves from your nostrils towards the point where your eyes are focused. (Do not stare at this point. Just allow your eyes to be softly focused there. To help with this, imagine that the focus is actually one inch above the ground where you are looking. This is the point at which you allow the air to dissolve.)

The half-Lotus meditation pose.

STEP 5: We first begin with concentration on this process. To do this, let the air come in and as it goes out allow the out breath to be given the number "one." The air comes in, and the next breath out is "two." Repeat this process until the count of twenty-one. If your mind becomes distracted and you lose track of your count, go back to "one." Also, don't count in an automatic f..shion. The important thing is for your mind to be focused and in sync with your body.

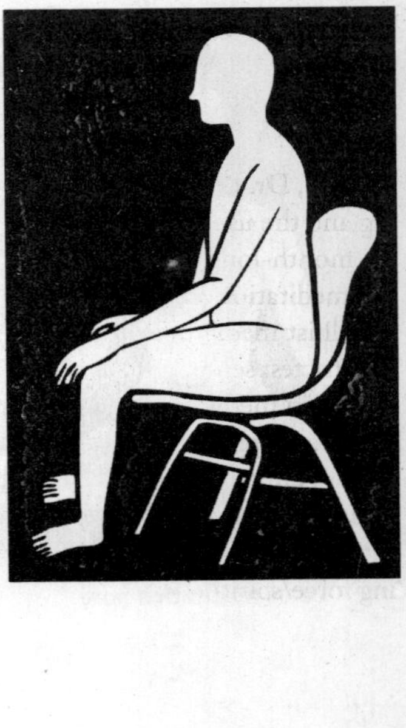

Meditation pose in a chair.

STEP 6: After counting to twenty-one, allow yourself to continue to pay attention to the out breath at the tip of your nostrils and the sense that the air dissolves into the space before you. If your mind drifts from attention on this, just say to yourself the word *thinking*. Then draw your attention back to your breath and carry on.

STEP 7: Allow yourself at least twenty minutes for this process. The time can then be expanded to forty minutes, then to one hour. The important point here is to be consistent with your practice. Short periods regularly will yield better results than long periods done erratically.

The goal of such meditation is to allow equanimity to arise naturally. One learns to give up fixation on various thoughts and feelings by experiencing how they come and go—as does the breath. As we see that this is true in our own lives, it becomes possible to see that it is also true for others. Knowing how easily we become fixated or addicted to this or that and the suffering that results, we wake up to the suffering of others and see them in a new way. In this manner we can give up guilt and blaming and get in touch with the basic goodness that is our nature and the nature of others. In deepening this experience, compassion and genuine caring for others naturally arises.

HEALING MEDITATION

In 1988, Dr. Lobsang Rapgay gave a day-long seminar on healing and the use of meditation in the healing process as a part of his month-long training program in San Francisco. The healing meditation presented is similar in format to other Tibetan Buddhist meditation practices. Although not a visualization in the strictest sense, it is based on a time-tested formula for the best results in meditation and healing rituals. If you are not using a traditional practice, this formula gives you a means of creating a more effective ritual of healing meditation for your situation. This format is based on the dignity and etiquette of "civilized" interaction. In this case your interaction is with whatever healing force/spirit/deity you identify with. You contemplate why you want to be in this healer's presence and be healed by him or her; visualize the healer before you and make efforts to establish a contact; arrange to meet and establish a sense of the healer's presence and of yourself being in his or her presence; praise the healer's healing qualities and abilities as you would complement an honored guest; make your request; be willing to experience any procedure the healer wants you to go through; and, finally, thank him or her for coming. Of course, in the tradition of Tibetan medicine and Buddhist ethics, altruism is a sign of healthy intention; you also want others to be healed and hope that whatever healing you receive may also benefit others.

The following meditation narrative can initially be read so that you can familiarize yourself with the sequence. You may want to create a more personalized version by making a tape recording, providing gaps in the sequence so you have time to work with the visualization and have time for the healing interaction to take place. Although the session can be designed for whatever time period you feel comfortable with, ideally you should take a minimum of twenty minutes. And, like sitting meditation, short sessions on a daily or regular basis are better than doing sporadic meditation marathons. Such an approach is crisis management and will usually not be as effective as a more consistent effort. Sound prevention comes from the building of good, consistent habits.

The healing meditation presented here is divided into three parts.

Part one involves creating a sense of deep relaxation on the levels of body, speech, and mind by using isometrics, specific breathing rhythms, and the repetition of certain sounds to be said silently in our minds.

Part two is a contemplative exercise. We try to see ourselves as we really are. We become aware of our own mortality by reflecting on birth, sickness, old age, and death itself. We also look at our minds. We look at our vulnerability on a basic level, recognizing the fragileness of our lives and various conditions that impinge on our very existence as well as the impact of society and other factors on our well-being. Here we also cultivate an existential awareness of the inherent loneliness of human existence and how intensely dependent we are on our world and its various conditions.

Part three is a step-by-step process to develop freedom from these conditions by working with the healing process that brings us in touch with our true nature. This process involves letting go of dependency on external conditions, objects, persons, and so forth. We attempt to come to the realization that loneliness and the dark forces that we experience are vehicles for us to appreciate who we are and recognize our connection to that which is around us. We look to our own potentials in order to become independent.

As we contemplate and meditate with such understanding, we relax more with who we are. Being less agitated, we are less caught up in past, present, and future. Nowness brings about the balanced working between mind and body. This is where true healing becomes possible.

Part One

STEP 1: Sitting on a cushion so that your crossed legs allow your knees to be below the level of your navel, breathe in a natural manner so that your diaphragm is relaxed and your belly is able to rise and sink with each breath. Rest your hands on your knees so that your ring fingers rest in the hollow on the outside of your kneecaps; this activates the energy of what is known as the Wisdom Channel. Allow your tongue to rest towards the front of the arch on your upper palate.

STEP 2: Breathe in and out fully and deeply three to five times.

STEP 3: Tense and relax each of the following areas three times each. After performing the isometric three times for a given area of the body, take three relaxing breaths before going to the next area mentioned.

a. Breathe in, hold the breath, and tense the feet for a moment; then breathe out and let go of the tension. Repeat this two more times for a total of three repetitions. (Follow this same procedure for each area that is mentioned.)
b. the calves
c. the abdomen (Here you want to draw up the muscles of the groin as well.)

d. the arms and hands (The fingers here are outstretched.)
e. the jaw (Here you are clenching the teeth.)

STEP 4: Then silently to yourself, using the following breathing sequence with sounds

a. Breathe in, saying silently to yourself the sound "OM" (pronounced as AUM)
b. Holding the breath for a moment, say to yourself "AH"
c. Breathe out while saying to yourself the sound "HUNG" (pronounced HOONG)
d. Repeat the sequence three, five, seven, or twenty-one times.

STEP 5: After doing these sounds internally, rest your attention on your breath. Watch the stream of your breath as it comes into your body, down into your relaxed stomach to a point about one and one-half inches below your navel, and then moves out of your body past the tip of your nose. Feel that the breath stream leaves the tip of your nose and dissolves in a space that is six feet in front of you on the ground. Continue to observe your breath in this manner for five minutes.

Parts Two and Three

The remaining portions are combined in the following sequence:

1. Contemplating your purpose and intention for doing the meditation
2. Visualizing the image of your ideal healer
3. Seeking permission from the healer
4. Experiencing satisfaction
5. Interaction with the healer
6. Developing self-confidence and independence
7. Thanksgiving

Although the technique presented here is generic, its format is similar to the strict forms of the various meditations in Tibetan Buddhist tradition, including that of the Medicine Buddha. The length of time for doing this practice can range from twenty minutes to any desired time.

STEP 1: Contemplating your purpose and intention for doing the meditation. Why are you doing this practice? As you sit quietly, contemplate what you need to work on to manifest healthiness. Think on all levels of your existence: physical, psychological/emotional, spiritual. Once you've established what needs to be addressed, the purpose is to focus on healing that condition.

Initially you may be focusing on yourself, but to make your motivations for healing totally pure, you must also recognize the suffering of others. Seeing the suffering that all beings experience, create the intent to not only do this healing meditation for yourself but also for the benefit of others. Your pain is just part of the greater pain experienced by others.

STEP 2: Visualizing the image of your ideal healer. Once you have figured out what it is that you need to work on, contemplate the ideal healer with whom you wish to interact. Is it the Medicine Buddha? Is it Jesus? Is it healing spirit or energy that you have a strong connection with? Establish an image of the healer with whom you want to interact and visualize that healer clearly in front of you, slightly above the level of the horizon.

STEP 3: Seeking permission from the healer. Like making an appointment to see a revered physician, you want to connect with the healer. Seek permission from your healer to interact with him/her to receive positive energies for yourself and others. It is in the act of including others in your request that permission is granted. (What you are practicing here is a very respectful and mature approach to the situation. You are taking ordinary day-to-day social skills and putting them to use in your spiritual practice. In fact, all tantric meditational practices utilize civilized social skills as a means of creating a sane and balanced approach to working with spiritual forces. This, in turn, has a way of uplifting all of our daily interactions.)

STEP 4: Experiencing satisfaction. Having made a proper connection with your healer and received permission to interact with him/her, you experience a sense of happiness. Allow yourself to feel this genuinely before you continue.

STEP 5: Interaction with the healer. Basically you are committing yourself to the prescription of the healer. You look to the healer, and the healer sends out rays of white light from his/her heart in all directions simultaneously. This light is received by all the enlightened beings of all directions. As they receive this they know that you are doing this healing practice with pure motivation. In response, they send back multicolored, and especially dark blue, light which enters into the heart of the healer. Now the healer is more powerful than before. He/she embodies the energy and healing power of all enlightened beings.

As you now breathe in, you see that from the heart of the healer light rays flow and enter into your nostrils. (For a LUNG or TRIPA rang-zhin or condition, the basic healing color is dark blue. If your condition is more BEKAN, you want the light to be reddish white.) This light goes into your nostrils and goes through your entire system but especially to areas where you are experiencing pain or stress. The colored light then dissolves the pain or stress into small dark particles which leave your nostrils as you breathe out like smoke and dissolve back into the natural elements in the ground before you, where they can create no more harm.

Breathe in and out like this three, seven, or twenty-one times. Then focus your attention on other beings. See in front of you those with whom you have personal difficulties, friends behind you, and others to your sides. See the light from the healer pouring from his/her heart and entering and cleansing all others as was done for you. See this happening three, seven, or twenty-one times.

STEP 6: Developing self-confidence and independence. You are now transformed, not vulnerable as before. You are more assured, self-confident. You are freed of distraction and no longer trapped by circumstances or projections. You experience independence and your true strength.

As you experience these qualities in your being, you see that the healer before you is more at a distance. He/she now stands as a witness. What has been given to you is nothing more than your true nature, but now no longer veiled. Thus you are no longer in a state of dependence.

STEP 7: Thanksgiving. At this point, you express gratitude to the healer and others for their help. Proper motivation here is the wish that whatever benefit you have received may be extended to all sentient beings who experience pain and suffering. With this thought and sense of gratitude, you now allow the image of the healer to dissolve back into the emptiness from which it arose.[1]

INDIVIDUAL SPIRITUAL ORIENTATION

In 1988, Sangye Wangchuck, a Bhutanese astrologer, presented material on various aspects of Tibetan astrology to a seminar at Matrix Software in Big Rapids, Michigan. Sangye discussed one of the key aspects of this astrological system called *mewas.* Roughly translated, the word *mewa* means "blemish" or "birthmark." These mewas correlate to the yin and yang aspects of the transformative energies presented in the Chinese Law of Five Transformations. Further information regarding the theory behind the mewas and the Law of Five Transformations can be found in my book *The Complete Guide to Nine-Star Ki,* which delves into a system of astrology found in Tibet, China, Japan and intimated in the Vedic astrology of India.[2]

Briefly summarized, each year is governed by a particular mewa. The mewa of the year that you were born into has a profound influence on how you conduct your life most effectively. In his presentation, Sangye Wangchuck focused on how the mewa associated with one's year of birth creates a certain type of orientation in spiritual life. Specific Buddhist deity meditations were given, meditations that help people to focus on the cultivation of the qualities that will lead them rapidly along in their spiritual development. Some people need meditations on equanimity, some on purification; some need to feel enriched, others need to feel a connection with ancestry.

In *The Complete Guide to Nine-Star Ki,* this material is presented in such a way that readers will know the most useful direction in which to orient themselves in their spiritual endeavors. While the specific deity practices of the Buddhist tradition have been eliminated, the qualities embodied by that deity remain the focus of the narrative. Those wanting the original transcripts with this information as presented by Sangye

Wangchuck, should contact Matrix Software in Big Rapids, Michigan (see Resources for address).

There are nine mewas. The symbolism ascribed to each mewa is a number, one through nine, a color, and an element or transformation phase. These are a form of shorthand indicating particular physical, psychological, and spiritual predispositions. The spiritual aspect of each one of these mewas is presented below in nine narratives. To find out which narrative relates to you, find your birth year on the chart provided in the final chapter, "Time and Place."

ONE White Water

Because of their deep spiritual nature, it is *meaning* that plays a central role in the spiritual life of ONE White Waters. Events of life come fast and furious to these people, and it is the challenge for them to learn and let go almost simultaneously.

To "be here now," these people need to go through some form of purification process, like a baptism—to clear things out and develop the ability to let go of what must be released. Humor is an attribute to cultivate since it is easy for such people to be overly serious about the significance of everything and hold onto issues unnecessarily. As they let go and "go with the flow," their insights become easier to communicate rather than being deep, dark secrets.

Because of their depth and sensitivity, such people have an innate sense of the human condition. Although they can act condescendingly toward others, much of this behavior comes from caring too much for others. With more detachment, this way of being that creates barriers between themselves and others can be transformed into an active compassion that will be like soothing waters to those other people.

Relaxation exercises and silent meditations are helpful for these types. Periods of retreat are also useful, provided they do not feel isolated. Having bowls of water on a shrine is grounding, as is the use of sound, especially chimes and crystal bowls or gongs. Meditations on compassion should be emphasized. As sexuality can be an important factor in their spiritual development,

ONE White Waters who have done purificatory practices and have some mental stability in meditation may wish to investigate the Tao of Love or consult with an authentic master regarding tantric sexual practices.[3]

TWO Black Earth

Service to others is the hallmark of TWO Black Earth people. And to allow this virtue to arise more out of altruism, they need to address self-doubt and a deep sadness that they often harbor. These two factors, if allowed to cloud their worldview may create cynicism, contempt for others, or jealousy. Thus such people need to work on cultivating greater confidence in themselves.

To accomplish this, TWO Black Earth people should find others who have committed themselves to the spiritual values and path they wish to follow. Because of their devotional nature and team mentality, they can be examples of religious/spiritual discipline to others. At the same time, such people need to be very conscious of being able to distinguish between faith and blind adherence.

Compassion is strong in such people, yet they need to understand the difference between true compassion and what the great Tibetan master, the Venerable Chogyam Trungpa, Rinpoche, calls "idiot compassion," or codependence. Rather than just giving due to a feeling of obligation, they must pay more attention to what the real need of the situation is in order to truly be beneficial in their service and to avoid being rebuffed more than appreciated for what they do.

Self-empowerment practices and meditations are advised. The use of music and chanting in this context are useful. Once they have overcome doubt, and thus become confident in their service and compassion, the unconditional nature of the TWO Black Earth people can be a powerful force in clearing away obstacles in life for themselves and others around them.[4]

THREE Blue Space

The main issues in the spiritual life of THREE Blue Space people are grounding and maturation. Such people have a natural experience of spaciousness in their way of being, along with an intensity which can be inhibiting to those around them. Developing greater sensitivity to others and learning how to ground this energy will help in all circumstances.

As their power of seeing, both in a mundane but also spiritual sense, presents them with a vivid picture of whatever aspect of reality they are focusing on, any spiritual practice that involves visualization will be excellent in channeling and grounding the intensity of such people. At the same time, because of their natural experience of space, meditations of a Zen nature that emphasize the insubstantial nature of phenomena, the breath, even space itself, are useful. Sacred sound or mantra is beneficial for these people as it can channel the tremendous energy they carry in their voices. Other meditative practices and disciplines that have as their focus purification will help such people ground and clarify their actions, speech, and mental patterns.

What these people must guard against in considering all of the practices mentioned is constantly changing and mixing them up, thus diluting their effectiveness. Their interests are so broad that rather than go deep and experience the fruition of spiritual practices, such types may spread themselves too thin to accomplish much in any particular direction. If they allow themselves to go deeper, such people will be able to develop their mystic nature, the primary expression and strength underlying their spiritual qualities.[5]

FOUR Green Space

FOUR Green Space people are excellent generalists, but to get a better perception of reality, they need to develop their potential for penetration. From the space quality of their mewa, it is as if they get a good sense of what is going on around them but need to allow their vision to deepen beyond first impressions. These people possess a natural impatience which pushes them ahead to the next thing; thus what is presently around them is felt, but somewhat unclearly. If they pause, look more deeply, and get a better perspective, their actions in the moment are magnetizing and rich. From another aspect of their mewa, associated with wood or trees, they are like the first shoots of young saplings that break through the ground in early spring. All of the environmental elements of wind, sun, water, and so on hit them for the first time. They are aware of everything that is impacting them and are quite vulnerable to this stimulation, but need to get greater clarity about what is really happening to them and those around them. Thus they need to cultivate patience, something that can be a potent antidote to their tendency to be bored or frustrated.

"Cleanliness is next to godliness" is a useful dictum for FOUR Green Space people. They need to take care of their own cleanliness and the cleanliness of their environment. For only in a serene environment can they experience the space they need to tame a frenetic churning that enters their lives in the midst of chaos. In such a serene atmosphere they penetrate deeper into life's mysteries and thus cultivate an inner strength that can prevent them from being sidetracked or overwhelmed because of their sensitivity.

It is wise for FOUR Green Space persons to seek out a teacher with whom they feel a kinship. Meditation where movement is involved (i.e., tai chi, yoga) is also advantageous.[6]

FIVE Yellow Earth

Tibetan tradition views people with the FIVE Yellow Earth mewa as the most naturally religious people. There is a strong link between them and their ancestors, and thus they should make the veneration of ancestors a part of their spiritual life, including any lineage of teachers or teachings they may align themselves with.

FIVE Yellow Earth people have very deep longings when it comes to their spiritual life. Yet, because they are quick to think and act, such people may miss opportunities for growth and learning if they are not obvious. To deepen their understanding, they must therefore develop better listening skills and take time for contemplation. Stillness is needed to balance their restless nature. Since FIVE Yellow Earth people thrive with music around them, the use of ritual music and chanting are useful in nurturing their spiritual development. Such practices can prevent them from excessive self-involvement and concern.

These people are naturally altruistic, yet at the same time stoic and, at times, gruff. Their altruism often goes unnoticed because they will usually find an unusual, but often perfect solution to a problem. Consequently, others may reject their offers of help or not fully appreciate what FIVE Yellow Earth people have done for them. Of all the numbers, they are the most misunderstood and disliked just for being themselves. Such people are advised to cultivate the virtues of patience, tolerance, and humility to soften their character and help ameliorate the difficulties that may arise between themselves and others.[7]

SIX White Air

SIX White Air people have powerful psychic abilities and intuitive awareness. These types also have a strong sense of morality and a need for social structure and community mores. Because they view historical factors as important, they usually align themselves to a tradition that has a legitimate social or cultural basis.

If dietary and lifestyle factors lead them to be imbalanced in one direction, they may overemphasize psychic abilities and lose their grounding and connection with everyday life. On the other hand, if they become too rigid in diet and lifestyle, they may ignore their intuitive sensibility and plunge into ardent dogmatism. By maintaining a balanced lifestyle they can develop a strong, well-defined foundation for their religious or spiritual life—one that will allow their minds to explore areas that others are not sensitive to. By balancing their intuition with their connection to society, their deeper intuitive knowledge can become a wellspring from which they can work towards peace and universal brotherhood. SIX White Airs will find it more comfortable to meditate in a group, rather than alone.

SIX White Airs should make a point of acknowledging the importance of their environment and ancestry. This serves as protection in their spiritual growth and expression. Such people are also naturally inclined towards philanthropic gestures, as long as they feel that what they are contributing to is beneficial to society.[8]

SEVEN Red Air

The I Ching trigram for SEVEN Red Air is the Joyous Lake (Tui). Like a calm, cool lake, SEVEN Red Air people are characterized by a gentle, calm exterior concealing a strong, deep interior.

These people can appear calm on the surface and have the capacity to reflect whatever is around them. Although such reflections may only be superficial, SEVEN Red Air people can get quite preoccupied with such appearances, like being involved with a mirage. They may even recognize at some level that what they are preoccupied with is only superficial but because they get caught up in the excitement of an experience, the deeper meanings may elude them. The more preoccupied they become, the more they are like a lake that has become turbulent. They then see only distortions and can appear quite groundless, immersing themselves in experiences just for the sake of having them.

SEVEN Red Air people thus must be aware of the tendency to develop addictive attitudes. In order to help counteract this tendency, they should cultivate time and space for solitude. Breathing-style meditations are useful to calm the mind and body. Once the lake is allowed to calm down, the reflection on the surface can then be contemplated and evaluated, and what is below the surface can be viewed more clearly. Then SEVEN Red Air people can bring up from their depths awarenesses and perceptions that may have been hidden from themselves as well as others. Although they may express these awarenesses in somewhat intellectual or metaphysical terms, the SEVEN Red Air people who give themselves time to drink from their own depths can experience a lasting sense of joy.

Meditation practices that emphasize healing are particularly recommended.[9]

EIGHT White Earth

A natural tendency towards stillness and constancy that EIGHT White Earth people exhibit in their daily routines finds its highest expression in their creation of a peaceful and deep spiritual life. EIGHT White Earth people need to work on getting a larger view of the workings and nature of things around them rather than the minute details. The details are easy for them to focus on, but if they become too obsessed with such details they may not see "the forest for the trees." They are of particular service to others when they can find pragmatic ways of helping people with their problems. EIGHT White Earth people are quite private in their emotional expression and thus do not function well when much emotion is expressed towards them or demanded from them. Such people have strong faith that is demonstrated by the acts they perform.

EIGHT White Earth people will find spiritual contemplation easier in clean, orderly environments. A shrine or altar showing respect for earthly forces and elements is helpful. Gaining a wider view and relating to the beauty of nature in their meditations can counteract their tendency to make everything solid in their lives, including their notion of self, and thus help to lighten their load. For these people spiritual life need not be serious and intense to be well considered.[10]

NINE Maroon Fire

As fire lights up the dark revealing what is present, so NINE Maroon Fire people have the potential for discriminating awareness. Also, just as fire reveals both an object and its shadow, NINE Maroon Fire people may find themselves better able to identify both obvious and underlying meanings than those around them. (However, these people may lack discretion when sharing their insights with others. They have a tendency to be painfully blunt.) Rooted on the earth and reaching towards heaven, NINE Maroon Fire people have a very direct approach to spiritual matters. Even the most profound esoteric truths may be obvious facts for them. In NINE Maroon Fire people, this is compounded by the fact that they have clairvoyant abilities and thus are aware of the invisible world around them more than others.

Thus these people can be a light for themselves and—due to the power of their charisma—for those around them. What they must guard against is being caught up in their own emotions, which can be quite passionate. Such passion can sometimes blind them, especially when what is being examined is personal. They should attempt to temper their tendency to get caught up in appearances and allow their minds to focus more intensely on what they are perceiving. By developing their discriminating awareness, they will thus have clearer perceptions, have better intuitive judgment about sharing what they are seeing, and will speak with more intellectual clarity.[11]

For further information about Tibetan astrology, Windhorse Imports in the United Kingdom can put people in touch with expert Tibetan astrologers in India who do astrological charts specifically on spiritual issues and useful life practices (see Resources).

DEALING WITH PROBLEMS ARISING IN MEDITATION

As mentioned previously meditation is an active process, a process of being present and allowing our sense of separation from the world to dissolve. Our limited views stifle our natural potentials, and by cutting through these we become more empowered. However, empowerment is not about "me" becoming powerful. Empowerment occurs when the "me" that causes separation from anything not "me" dissolves and the flow of energy that exists within and without oneself is experienced as one. In the Buddhist tradition, this is sometimes referred to as the experience of "one taste."

Of course, the ego doesn't particularly like this. This change of views and fixations is often a very painful process. Sometimes we experience physical pain, sometimes emotional, even spiritual pain. Shambhala Training master Chogyam Trungpa, Rinpoche, uses the analogy that it is like trying to emerge from a cocoon as a butterfly.[12] Unlike the natural process of becoming a butterfly, however, there is no particular guarantee that our spiritual growth will follow a set or predictable pattern. In the process of spiritual development, when all else fails to stop the progress of ego dissolution, self-denigration, the ultimate ego trick, can keep us in our place, making us only conscious of our limitations rather than our potentials.

Distractions, pain, and confusion arise in meditation as we learn to discipline our minds and to let go of what arises in our experience. As we become more adept at remaining in meditative equipoise, such pains and distractions can come and go without any particular intervention. They even become inspirational as we see them for what they are.

However, there are times when we become thoroughly distracted by a pain, an emotion, a thought, or some level of torpor or dullness of mind. To deal with these situations, the following antidotes are provided. (Each antidote offered is complete in itself. These are not series. However, you may find that in different circumstances, one antidote works better than another.) Although they come from various sources, particular credit is given here to Venerable Khenpo Karthar, Rinpoche, Chime Rinpoche, Dr. Lobsang Rapgay, and Lama Ole Nydahl.

Dullness of Mind

1. Keep your eyes open while meditating; lift your gaze.
2. Lift your gaze to the level where the wall meets the ceiling, allowing your eyes to pan back and forth for a few minutes. Then bring your gaze back to the normal position. (This technique is especially good if you are sleepy.)
3. Imagine that an enlightened being (i.e., Buddha) that is very heavy is sitting one and one-half inches above your head.
4. For a few minutes, contemplate something that brings you joy, creating a positive intensity. Once your mind feels uplifted, resume meditation.

Distraction

1. If you are distracted by the room around you, close your eyes to meditate. If you are distracted by mental images when your eyes are closed, meditate with your eyes open. Ideally, the best position for the eyes is where they are one-quarter open.
2. Use breath as the object of meditation, mixing mind with space through breath.
3. Imagine that an enlightened being that is two inches tall is four feet away from you and looking directly into your eyes.
4. Imagine that a small black pea is in the ground just underneath where you sit. As your breath goes out, imagine that the stream of breath is traveling down into that black pea.
5. Contemplate something that moves you emotionally. This will help to ground you and bring you back to your body (calming LUNG). Resume meditation.

Getting Spaced Out

Mix a small amount of asfoetida (also known as hing) and ginger powder into some ghee. Warm this mixture and with your finger massage this mixture up into your nostrils until your eyes begin to tear.

Dizziness, Palpitation, Vomiting, Shooting Pains

Such symptoms can occur for any number of reasons, such as improper diet, excessive nervous tension, or worry. Try to contemplate what may be going on in your life. If, on the other hand, such symptoms occur with any frequency, discontinue meditation until you can get formal instruction from a meditation master.

Occasional Shooting Pains

Massage sesame oil into your ears, on the crown of your head, fontanelle points, temples, and occipital crest marma points.

Lights Flashing and Starry Formations Before the Eyes

This is a LUNG-TrIPA condition. Massage the following points around the eyes in the order suggested.→

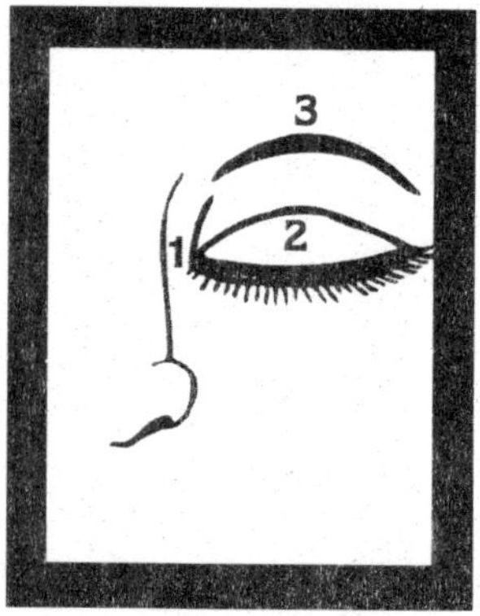

POINT 1—Press to the inside of the tear ducts.

POINT 2—Press on the upper portion of the eye and eyelid.

POINT 3—Press on the point in the middle and slightly above the eyebrow.

Pains in the Chest When Visualizing Mantras at the Heart

Energy in the sacred subtle channels is moving the wrong way. Discontinue visualization practice until you get more formal instruction from a meditation master.

Negative States of Mind

Untamed or non-transformed emotional states that create further confusion or suffering are called mental defilements or obscurations (in Tibetan *Klesas*). The following is a discussion of the psychological orientation one may adopt in the practice of meditation in order to assist in temporarily dispelling these negative states of mind.

For **Desire**, meditate on impermanence. Tibetans used to go to charnel grounds and meditate on skeletons. We can meditate on the experience of our heart pumping blood that is gushing through the body, or some other function of our own body.

Aggression/Anger is considered the worst of the mental obscurations as it inhibits spiritual development and weakens self-worth. An antedote to this emotional state is to meditate on loving kindness and patience (not dissimilar in effect from the practice of counting to ten). Time and space are often most useful for dealing with one's own anger as well as that of others. We should show compassion to others who are displaying anger.

Sometimes anger can be so intense that it allows no mental space to meditate. In this case get up from meditation and do something positive/beneficial. Arrange flowers on a shrine; do something useful for yourself or others. In this way you may lessen the effect of anger by not reinforcing it.

For **Ignorance**, you need to dispel resistance to change. Meditate on the breath, counting to twenty-five. Breathe in (one), out (two), in (three), and so forth. Watch your breath, the rhythm of breath, and the movement of your belly. Then relax your mind and observe the way your breath changes from moment to moment. This process creates lightness and mobility which overcome BEKAN qualities.

For **Jealousy**, meditate on generosity.

For **Pride**, the great Indian saint Nagarjuna teaches that one needs to become aware of one's insignificance. Go to a mountain and look over a valley. Or go into a crowd and experience yourself in the sea of humanity.

Please be aware that the practices suggested here are not exhaustive. Many great meditation masters offer alternative solutions or means to alleviate negative states of mind and overcome mental and physical destractions. Refer to the *Bibliography* for other sources.

chapter six

DETOXIFICATION AND REJUVENATION

Detoxification is an essential part of quality preventive health care. However, it is also both the most underestimated and abused process in its modern Western application. In Western conventional allopathic tradition, it is veritably ignored as a factor in health care. Common problems such as colds, flus, digestive upsets, and headaches are often signals that detoxification is warranted. But too often medical practitioners recommend and people use medications to mask or eliminate their discomfort from these symptoms rather than address root causes. This can make the problem worse and lead to chronic, even degenerative disease, the prescription for which is stronger medication or surgery. On the other side of the spectrum are health-conscious people who place too much emphasis on detoxification—on totally fat-free diets, bowel cleansers, excessive exercise regimens, an abundance of colonics, and so forth. Done properly, and in accordance with a person's constitution and current condition, all these procedures can be quite helpful. Cleaning out is useful. However, once cleaned out sufficiently, one needs to know how to renutrify and rejuvenate the body. Too often alternative health-care practitioners and lay people know how to eliminate the toxins but do not know how to rebuild. In fact, where there is chronic weakness and lassitude, detoxification may have the effect of exacerbating a condition, leaving a person even more vulnerable. In such cases, a person often needs to renutrify, to build themselves up to a stronger level, before a good detoxification process can be utilized effectively.

Just as detoxification is often misunderstood or misapplied, so is rejuvenation. To be youthful or vital in one's state of mind is universally considered a worthy and reachable goal. But while some people think the idea of retaining or regaining a youthful body a pipe dream, and others regard it as a goal worth religiously pursuing, still others view it as a denial of our inevitable biological demise. Although the Western medical model views rejuvenation as unscientific, this does not stop people from attempting it. And because so many try, there are plenty of pundits of beauty and health pushing products with claims far in excess of their actual benefits.

According to the Ayurvedic tradition of India and Tibet, and the Taoist system of China (which shows striking similarity in its approaches to the energetics of the body in advanced Tibet yogic practices) slowing down or reversing the aging process is possible. The highest purpose of the techniques employed is to retain youthful vigor so that one can maximally use this life for self-actualization and spiritual development. To employ these techniques to retain physical beauty or have a longer sex life is considered vain and pointless. Still, such techniques do have their more mundane purposes; for example, virilification to ensure that one produces appropriate progeny (usually sons) was traditionally used to carry on bloodlines in families.

Youthful strength and clarity to develop wisdom and compassion are aids to development of our human potential. However, even if one is physically ill and debilitated, such fine qualities can be developed. The mental and spiritual traits of wisdom and compassion far outshine physical perfection. And without development of spiritual capacities, a longer, more youthful life may be a waste of time. Indeed, the Venerable Chogyam Trungpa once said that if we were given a lifespan of a thousand years, with no clear spiritual development most of us would commit suicide by the age of three hundred.[1] Unless there is real mental and spiritual growth, the ability to preserve our flesh for eternity would only make us prisoners of the nightmare of old habitual patterns.

LEN NGA (Pancha Karma) THERAPY

Detoxification and rejuvenation are most effective when carried out in accordance with a person's constitution. Towards this end, the Ayurvedic traditions of India and Tibet have utilized a process called Len Nga (Tibetan) or Pancha Karma (Sanskrit). Translated, this means five *(Nga, Pancha)* actions *(Len, Karma)*.

According to Ivy Blank, former codirector of the Ayurvedic Center of Santa Fe, New Mexico,

> Pancha Karma (Len Nga) is a method developed by the ancient sages of Ayurveda for completely and scientifically purifying the human body of morbid substances, toxins, and accumulated wastes, and for rejuvenation through the administration of revitalizing substances and practices. This process helps people become more fit to accomplish their life tasks with strength, enthusiasm, and happy minds.[2]

This being said, the application of Len Nga is not restricted to spiritual seekers only. The *Charak Samhita*, the main treatise from which Ayurveda of today draws its information and practices, gives practical guidance in using Len Nga for specific illness, as a yearly cleansing and rejuvenative process, or in a spiritual context. For almost every illness suffered by humanity, there are Len Nga procedures and regimens; readers are encouraged to seek out a competent practitioner of Ayurveda for such information (see Resources).

Even though Len Nga offers considerable physical benefits, because of the psychological and spiritual orientation of Tibetan medicine, Dr. Lobsang Rapgay emphasizes the use of Len Nga therapy for psychological and spiritual transformation. The detoxifying and rejuvenating aspects of Len Nga therapy create a deep state of true relaxation as well as greater body agility and are useful for mind/body transformation. But even more profound is the way in which Len Nga opens the door for personal exploration and growth towards a more awakened state of being.

The Techniques

Before specifying how each nyepa type can utilize Len Nga therapy, a general description of the techniques employed is useful.

Len Nga actually is the five processes that deeply detoxify the body. These are enemas, purgatives, emesis (vomiting), nasal administration, and blood and nerve cleansing. These five are the core techniques utilized. However, there are other techniques applied prior to and/or in conjunction with these techniques.

Some are preparatory and almost always applied while others relate to specific conditions and are only used when appropriate.

Unless you know your rang-zhin and how your current condition affects your constitution, an initial evaluation is first necessary. This will determine how Len Nga therapy will be practiced.

Once a date has been established for therapy to begin, preparatory lifestyle changes are encouraged. A few days before starting therapy, diet should be modified. One eliminates all raw foods, alcohol, juices, caffeinated drinks, and meat from daily consumption. Traditionally a meal call *kichadi* is recommended. Made of white basmati rice, split mung beans, and spices, this provides enough sustenance to keep the body supplied with calories and nutrients while allowing the digestive system to calm down. This meal, along with steamed vegetables and mild herbal teas or hot water, is to be consumed prior to, during, and a few days following the Len Nga process. If the kichadi cannot be made, a basic, nonspicy vegetarian diet of grains and vegetables is suggested. An herbal intestinal cleanser called *trifala* may be started at this time. In some cases more specific herbal preparations for bowel cleansing are recommended.

Massage and Steam Hydrotherapy

The actual start of the Len Nga therapy is massage and hydrotherapy, usually in the form of herbal baths or steam. Depending on the constitution, various types and amounts of oils are used for massage. Generally, sesame oil is used because it is most effective in drawing out toxicity from the tissues and renutrifying the cells. Besides the traditional massage techniques of percussion, friction, and kneading, various points called marmas are stimulated. Literally translated, marma means a point that can kill. Indeed, some of the marmas have been identified in martial art traditions and are used combatively. The slightest touch to specific marmas can bring paralysis, even death. However, rest assured that these are not indicated or used in the massage procedures. Dr. Harish Johari in his *Ayurvedic Massage* identifies the marmas as neurolymphatic points. They help to stimulate the movement of lymph for the purpose of elimination as well as activating all of the organ systems of the body. Along with these marma points, special emphasis is placed on the joints and the abdomen. The greatest concentration of red blood cells is around the joints. Hence working on the joints helps to improve circulation and reoxygenate the blood. Working the abdomen thoroughly and applying heat there prepares the intestinal tract for the toxins released into the bloodstream and lymphatic system from the massage techniques. Thus more effective elimination is ensured.

Depending on the dominant nyepa, the emphasis in massage application will vary. For LUNG-types, slow, gentle, and consistent touch and pressure is recommended. Such people need to feel pacified and nurtured during the massage. TrIPA-types need work that is precise yet spacious. They can be the most talkative during the massage, asking what you are doing and why. Provide clear explanations yet constantly encourage them to relax. Concerning the marmas and acupuncture points (if used), rather than emphasizing the pressing in on a point focus on releasing it. BEKAN-types often fall asleep during massage. For them, strong stimulation is encouraged, but this does not mean that it is necessary to knead deeply. Rapid friction is very effective. Occasional unexpected movements or changing the sequencing of what you do can help to keep their attention and energy focused. Briefly, keep the LUNG-types quiet and warm, the TrIPA-types relaxed, and the BEKAN-types attentive.

The herbal bath or steam bath follows the massage. Some herbs are generally useful for all constitutions, such as bay, eucalyptus, and ginger. However, other herbs are used for specific effects. The primary intent of this process is to increase circulation and to allow the oils and herbs to penetrate deeply into the body for a more effective detoxification. Unlike a sweat lodge or steam room, the steam bath used is an individual process. Spa-type steam boxes are used so that the head stays cool—something that can be accomplished also by pouring water over the head or keeping it wrapped in a cool towel. With the head kept cool, the body can take more heat for a longer time, with fifteen to twenty minutes usually sufficient.

Following this procedure, the body is cleansed of whatever remaining oil is left on or just under the skin. This is done by rubbing the body down with a number of different grain or bean flours. Chickpea or garbanzo flour is generally used. The flour absorbs the oil, leaving the skin smooth and invigorated. It also ensures that the toxins released into the oil will be removed and not be remetabolized by the body. This prevents the body from feeling sore or sluggish the next day. Massage therapists should understand that the experience of tiredness and aching after massage is not necessarily a sign of detoxification but can be the result of retoxification if too much oil used is reabsorbed and the digestive tract is not prepared for toxins. The heat to the abdomen and flour cleansing technique utilized in the Len Nga preparatory massage ensure that these symptoms will not occur.

Although these techniques can be done generally for a pleasing, stress-reducing experience, massage and hydrotherapy are done daily during Len Nga therapy. When done daily for whatever time period therapy is to be engaged in, they have a more profound effect. Beyond the general effect of relaxation, are the deeper effects of reduction or elimination of chronic symptoms as well as an emotional release and deepened spiritual focus that creates the quality of a spiritual journey.

The Five Actions

Depending on a person's condition and nyepa type, one or more of the following procedures (technically called Len Nga, or the five actions) should be utilized along with the preparatory massage and hydrotherapy. The descriptions provided here include a sense of how the procedures or techniques are carried out and under what circumstances they are useful.

Digestive Cleansing

Each of the nyepas has a storehouse in the body. When the body is in balance, these storehouses are like batteries, storing the nyepa energy and ensuring that the tissues, organs, and fluids in the body requiring the energy from a given nyepa receive it. When out of balance, it is as though the batteries are leaking; energy seeps away from the storehouse and gets disproportionately distributed throughout the tissues, organs, and channels of the body. In Len Nga therapy, the purpose of massage and the hydrotherapy is to eliminate some of the excess unbalanced energy through the skin's pores and drive the remainder back into the storehouses where it can then be removed from the body via normal eliminative channels. Herbs may be used to facilitate this process.

What makes this a logical and suitable course for restoration and balance of the nyepas is that these storehouses, or seats, are situated in the digestive tract. The seat of LUNG is in the colon or large intestine. The seat of TRIPA is in the small intestine. The seat of BEKAN is the stomach. Effective elimination from these regions of the digestive tract requires specific techniques.

1. Enemas (Tibetan: **Jamtsi)**

Enemas are intended to cleanse and rejuvenate the large intestine. Therefore their primary intent is to restore the balance of LUNG in the body. Enemas are an essential treatment for LUNG-type constitutions and conditions.

In Western alternative health care, we look at enemas as being less therapeutic than colonics. Because water is used in colonics, they do a good job of clearing out old fecal matter blocking circulation and efficient elimination. However, water has a drying effect on the lining of the colon. The dryness created can actually aggravate LUNG. Thus for LUNG-types, the result may be increased gas and bloating. Unfortunately, many colon therapists view this as a sign that more colonics are indicated when the opposite is the case.

A variety of ingredients are used in Tibetan Ayurvedic enemas, or *jamtsi.* Primary ingredients include decoctions from herbs used to break down and dissolve old fecal matter and revitalize the colon, and oil, either sesame oil or ghee, to soothe the intestinal lining and reduce LUNG. Other ingredients can be salt, honey, and milk to name a few. Thus enemas are tailored to suit the client's needs—to be more cleansing, nutritive, or calming. An example of the latter is how enemas with calming herbs are used for treating persons experiencing psychotic episodes or extreme mental distress.[3]

Although we are talking here about enemas being a part of the Len Nga process, they can also be utilized whenever LUNG symptoms (such as gas, constipation, tension headaches) arise. They are best done between 4:00 and 7:00 A.M. or 4:00 and 7:00 P.M.

2. Purgation (Tibetan: Shel)

The small intestine is the seat of TRIPA, and primary Len Nga technique used for TRIPA-type constitutions and conditions are purgatives. Enemas work on the large intestine; purgatives work on the small intestine.

During oil massages and steaming, enemas are often done daily. This is not true for purgatives. Purgation *(shel)* is usually done once at the end of a given number of sessions. It is customary to prepare the body for several days before the purgation by having the client consume a small amount of ghee (clarified butter) on an empty stomach upon rising in the morning. The purgative substance itself can be any number of Ayurvedic herbal compounds. However, a strong decoction of senna tea or several tablespoons of castor oil are quite effective. The time of day to take such a purgative is about one to two hours after the midday meal (between 10 A.M. and 1 P.M.) or in the evening before retiring (10 P.M. to 1 A.M.).

Although enemas can be cleansing, nutrifying, or calming, the primary function of purgation is to be cleansing. After a few hours, during which time the person rests and refrains from eating, diarrhea will ensue. It will feel hot as it comes out. The stool may even have a light green or yellowish appearance. This is an indication that excess TRIPA is leaving the body via the rectum. What is interesting to note is that while diarrhea can generally feel draining, in the context of the Len Nga regimen, every bout of the diarrhea that comes out during purgation can make the person feel more alert, yet relaxed. The purge is complete when all that is coming out is a brackish-colored water.

Besides introducing purgation at a specific time in the Len Nga therapy, it can be useful during times when TRIPA symptoms arise such as migraines, nausea, and low-grade, persistent fevers. After a purgative is taken and evacuation has subsided, the reintroduction of food should be gradual and begin with bland foods such as soft and watery white basmati rice and well-steamed vegetables. A purgative challenges digestive fire (Tibetan: pho thut), thus a gradual build up to normal eating is recommended. For at least two to three days, continue bland foods and eat only when hungry. Avoid meat or raw juices during this time. Also, due to the strong nature of this treatment, basic contraindications for its use include pregnancy, hemorrhoids, and anemia. In addition, this treatment should not be used by people who are very young or very old.

3. Emesis, or Vomiting (Tibetan: **Kyuk)**

Like purgation, therapeutic vomiting *(kyuk)* is primarily for cleansing the body. And like a good purgative, the end result of therapeutic vomiting is increased energy.

Like purgation, emesis is a procedure used after a number of days of preparatory massage, steam, and possibly herbs and enemas. The focus of therapeutic vomiting is to eliminate excess BEKAN, usually in the form of congestion and excess mucus. The seat of BEKAN is in the stomach. Consequently, the expulsion of BEKAN is upwards through the mouth. The time of day for emesis should be midmorning (8 A.M. to 10 A.M.) when BEKAN is most dominant.

The following vomiting procedure is suggested by Ayurvedic physician Dr. Sunil Joshi:

Upon rising, make a light porridge from one tablespoon of whole wheat flour, ghee, a cup of water, and four teaspoons of raw sugar or ghur. This porridge is a way of activating stomach secretions in preparation for vomiting. One hour later, prepare a cup of tea brewed with one gram of calamus root powder, adding honey to taste after the tea has steeped. Allow this to settle in the stomach for about fifteen minutes. Then prepare a strong decoction of licorice tea. Use eighty grams of licorice root powder and about one quart of water. Drink as much of this as possible to expand the stomach.

Within approximately fifteen minutes spontaneous vomiting will ensue. Excess mucus gathered in the stomach and sinus cavities will come pouring out. If the emesis is successful, the net volume of what comes out will be greater than the volume of liquid and porridge you consumed. When you get to the point where bile is tasted, this is an indication that the excess BEKAN has been successfully removed.[4]

As should be obvious from the description, this is a very cathartic process and interestingly is not as uncomfortable as vomiting due to usual stomach or digestive upset. Rest is recommended afterwards. A gradual reintroduction of foods is also suggested, especially those that are light and warming. This is in keeping with dietary recommendations suggested for BEKAN-types and BEKAN conditions. Since the main elimination is mucus, early spring is the best time for emesis. Like enemas and purgatives, vomiting can be done separately from Len Nga therapy when BEKAN symptoms are present, such as allergic bronchial asthma, heaviness in the chest, colds, and some skin disorders. Contraindications include TB and pregnancy. As we are more BEKAN in our earlier years, children have a natural tendency to vomit with digestive upset. Thus, inducing emesis in children is not advised.

4. Nasal Therapy (Tibetan: Na Jong)

Air contains vital life force (Sanskrit: *prana*; Tibetan: *sok lung*) that is the subtle form of the LUNG nyepa. Since the nasal passages are the primary means through which this force enters the body, having them clean and capable of taking sok lung in more efficiently is a key to good health.

When our sinuses get blocked due to improper dietary practices, when our sense of smell is shocked by odors, or when we breathe erratically such as when emotionally upset or when having overexercised, the whole balance of life force in our body can be disrupted. Excess LUNG may become trapped in the head, making us feel spacey or out of sorts. Our moods may become affected. On a more physiological level our sinus cavities may show signs of stress, represented by dark curved lines under the eyes. According to Oriental visual diagnosis, this is also an indication of strain on the kidneys. To demonstrate the connection between nasal passages and the kidneys, inhale vigorously. Notice the drawing up effect in the middle region of the back over the kidneys. (This may illustrate why people who have habitually snorted cocaine end up with renal difficulties.)

Nasal administration utilizing oils, herbal powders, or smoke is called *Na Jong*. As a Len Nga therapy with the primary emphasis being on the subtle aspect of LUNG, it has benefits similar to enemas. Nasal administration of various medications can be cleansing, calming, or renutrifying. It "redirects body energy trapped in the throat, nose, sinuses, and head in general . . . effecting higher cerebral, sensory, and motor functions, including movement in the kidneys."[5]

Nasal administration Len Nga therapy is usually done at the end of massage and hydrotherapy. It may be done every day during Len Nga therapy or intermittently, depending on the needs of the client. At the same time, this therapy can be done by itself with beneficial results.

The following is a description of the procedure as taught by Melanie Sachs. She uses ginger juice and raw sugar in the Na Jong solution. The intent here is to clear the sinus passages, drive excess LUNG from the face and head, and to stimulate the kidneys. Please note the contraindications given.

Applied appropriately (Na Jong) is very useful; its effects run deep physiologically and emotionally. If applied inappropriately, it can disrupt body energy and uncomfortable symptoms can arise that may last a few days. Therefore, (Na Jong) should not be done after a bath, food, sex, consuming alcoholic beverages, during pregnancy or menstruation.

Equipment you will need

1. quarter of a cup of sesame oil (This is for when you are doing a facial-type massage not in conjunction with other preparatory Len Nga therapy.)
2. glass eye dropper with a rubber end
3. fresh ginger root
4. one teaspoon of raw brown sugar
5. a small amount of clean water
6. facial tissues
7. hot water bottle and hot water or a hot pack

Preparation

1. Grate the ginger using a fine grater. Squeeze out the juice into a small bowl. (One can also use a juicer if available.)
2. Add a pinch of brown sugar and a dash of water per two tablespoons of the ginger juice. The sugar stops the ginger from burning. (This solution should be stored in the refrigerator when not being used.)
3. Heat the water for the hot water bottle.
4. Warm the sesame oil.
5. Arrange all the equipment to be within easy reach.

Procedure

1. Have the client lie on their back.
2. (If not already done with preparatory Len Nga procedures) Give a vigorous facial massage with warm sesame oil. Clockwise circular motions will relieve stress in the facial tissues. However, the main point of the massage here is simply to increase circulation and work the oil into the skin.
3. Apply direct pressure to the sinuses along both sides of the nose and then above the eyes.
4. Place a facial tissue on both sides of the face so that the nose is the only exposed area. Lay the hot water bottle or hot pack on one side of the face for a short period of time and then repeat on the other side. (If using a hot water bottle, you may need to wrap it in cloth if it is too hot.) Keep applying heat in this way until the face is really rosy and the oil is but almost vanished from the surface of the skin.
5. Place a rolled-up towel under the neck of the client so that their head is supported but cocked; their nostrils pointing upwards.
6. While applying pressure to the left nostril with your own left index or middle finger, place three to five drops of the ginger juice mixture into the right nostril with the eye dropper. Massage the sinus areas above and below the right eye. The client's eye may tear, indicating some emotional release. They may also feel energy dancing over the face. Use smooth massage strokes to ground this energy. Ask the client when

they are ready for application to the left nostril. Proceed in the same manner as you did on the right side.

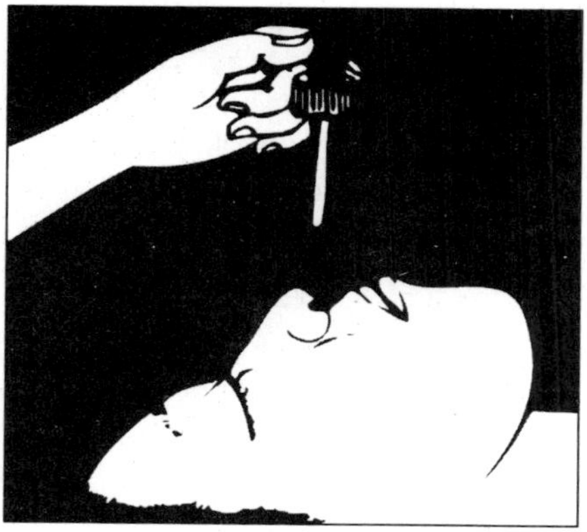

Drawing of a person receiving Na Jong.

7. Take your time. When the process is complete, support the client's shoulders as they sit up. Support the sternum with one hand and use your other hand to stroke down their spine. Have the client move slowly and suggest to them that they take their time with activities over the next hour.

> (Na Jong) can be done like this three days in a row. People report to me that after such a regimen they feel relaxed, sleep better, are more alert, and have more energy. The cheeks can become fuller and the sinus areas more open. It also releases tension in the neck. In such a short time, one may also observe a diminishing of rings below the eyes and an indication from the person that the condition of their kidneys has improved as they eliminate urine more efficiently.[5]

Other specific problems that nasal administration Len Nga also addresses are migraine, epilepsy, and ear and eye problems. The medications used for these problems will vary. One should consult a Tibetan or Indian Ayurvedic health practitioner when dealing with specific complaints.

5. Blood and Nerve Cleansing

Tibetan Ayurveda differs from Indian Ayurveda in this aspect of Len Nga therapy. In Indian Ayurveda, bloodletting is the fifth

Len Nga process. This technique is relegated to the third level of Tibetan medicine, considered as invasive as surgery. Such a process should only be done under the careful supervision of an Ayurvedic physician, and therefore, only a brief discussion of bloodletting is offered here.

A Tibetan lama visiting New Mexico once told a friend of mine how his father would periodically nick a blood vessel on the medial aspect of the heel of the foot in order to drain toxicity in the blood. At first the blood was dark; and when it became bright again, the procedure was finished and he would bandage the small incision. He and his friends would let blood especially when they had overindulged in eating and drinking.[7] In *Tibetan Buddhist Medicine and Psychiatry*, Terry Clifford writes of bloodletting's therapeutic use for demonic possession.[8] Thus this procedure is applied for physiological, psychological, and spiritual conditions. Ayurvedic physician Dr. Sunil Joshi speaks of its benefits for some skin diseases, headaches, and high blood pressure.[9]

The blood- and nerve-cleansing therapy listed as the fifth Len Nga therapy in the Tibetan tradition involves the use of herbs and inhaled substances to tonify the nerves and clean the blood. Blood conditions are often treated as a specific TRIPA problem since TRIPA is the nyepa that deals with the vascular system. Thus for cleansing purposes, TRIPA herbs and compounds, which are best prescribed by a competent Ayurvedic practitioner, are utilized. These herbs may be used in massage oil, in the steaming process, or as herbal tonics. This therapy is done in conjunction with other Len Nga therapies or may be used on an emergency basis when imbalances of blood and nerves are observed.

Among the five primary Len Nga therapies, there are many variations; and they can be applied in numerous ways. At the same time, along with these five, the two other Ayurvedic therapeutic procedures that follow are worth mentioning since they can be of tremendous benefit to people and are relatively easy and safe to administer.

NETRA BASTI

Netra Basti is a technique whereby the eyes are bathed in plain or medicated warm ghee. A ring of dough is built up around the eye to create a well, into which the ghee solution is poured. It is allowed to sit on the eye for approximately twenty minutes.

The Sanskrit word *basti* implies a cleansing action. Netra Basti is, therefore, a technique that has a cleansing effect on the eyes. Dust, dirt, even substances trapped in the eyes that a person has been unaware of can surface in the liquid ghee. Besides this cleansing aspect, Netra Basti is also nutritive. Gazing through a warm ghee solution has a directly nourishing effect on the optic nerve and the nervous system.

What follows is a description of how Netra Basti is performed. This technique can be used with Len Nga therapy as needed or in individual circumstances where it is deemed warranted. The lay person can experiment with this technique with very little concern for abreactions. Contraindications are active eye infections or conditions where surgery, medications, or other medical procedures have affected vision or the structure of the eye.

In order to perform Netra Basti you will need:

1. One cup of pure ghee, or clarified butter (This is easily made or purchased at an Indian or Oriental food store or natural food store.)
2. Whole wheat flour and water mixed to form a dough of earlobe consistency but slightly sticky, formed into a round doughnut-like ring big enough to encircle the eye
3. A quiet, warm, and tidy room that is pleasant smelling and pleasing to the senses

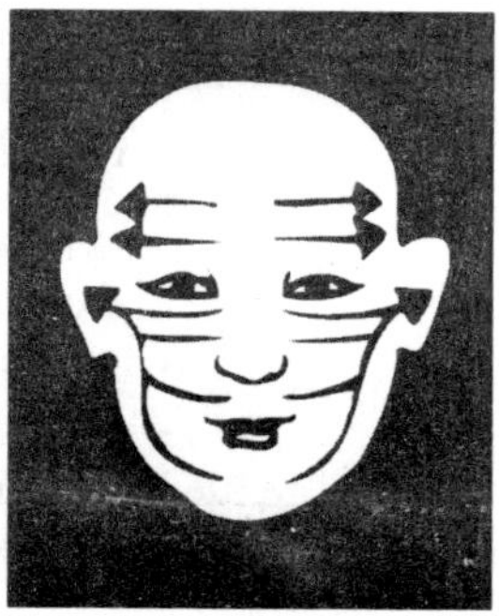

Massage prior to Netra Basti.

The person receiving the treatment needs to lie down on the back with the head and neck well supported. If this treatment is being done outside of the context of Len Nga preliminary therapies, give the face a firm yet gentle massage using stroking motions from the chin to the temples and then from the center of the forehead towards the ears.

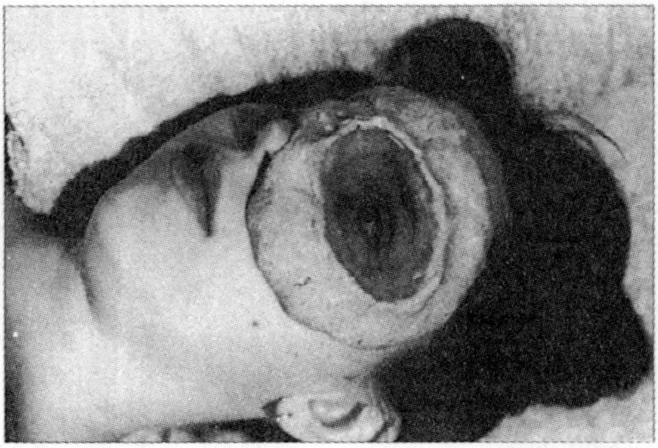

Dough ring around the eye acts as a well for the ghee.

Next, have the head slightly turned towards the left so that the right eye socket is facing the sky above. Apply the whole wheat doughnut around the right eye socket, pressing firmly to ensure that there is a good seal to the skin and the eye within the ring is able to open and close freely. You are basically creating a dough well around the eye into which the ghee solution will be poured.

Have the client close the right eye, and fill the dough cup with the ghee, which should be just slightly above room temperature. Pour slowly, starting at the corner of the eye so that the person can let you know how the temperature of the ghee feels. Once the eye is covered to the tips of the eyebrows, encourage the client to open and close that eye gently and slowly. The ghee should remain like clear amber liquid. If it begins to cloud or harden, it means that the ghee was at too low a temperature or that the room temperature is affecting the solidification. Ideally the ghee should remain clear for between fifteen to twenty minutes. It has been our experience that it is best to hold or at least make gentle contact with the head and neck during the treatment. As the ghee remains on the eye, physical and psychological changes can occur. The ghee can sting for a while as the eye releases tears and toxins, so the person should be reassured that this is a normal part of the process.

To remove the ghee, have the client tilt the head towards the right and allow the ghee to drain into a bowl. Do not reuse the ghee. Wipe the eye and the skin around the eye thoroughly. Repeat the process for the left eye. At the end of the session, it is also normal for the person to experience some blurriness of vision. If he or she plans to drive soon after the treatment, encourage the patient to wait about fifteen to twenty minutes.

In many circumstances, the author has been told by clients receiving Netra Basti of improvement in color perception and peripheral vision. In India, this therapy is used in the treatment of hyperactivity (attention deficit disorder) since Ayurvedic physicians believe this condition arises from the eye's inability to receive light properly. I have used this technique for such conditions, and parents have reported that their children slept better and were more focused as a result.

Netra Basti is also a treatment that can be used simply for beauty purposes. It brings a luster to the eyes, eliminates stress creases in the face, and can help to diminish bags under the eyes. Where eye strain arises from prolonged concentration (especially on computer terminals), Netra Basti can be a welcome treatment at the end of the day or week.

Case History

The following case history is used to demonstrate how this technique can be used in a more psychotherapeutic context:

Joyce was referred to me by a counselor, who felt that Joyce needed some massage work done to facilitate more emotional release for the counseling process. The primary technique I was to use was a Tibetan form of shiatsu or acupressure.

Joyce wore glasses, and it became readily apparent that there was a lot of tension around her eyes. After inquiring about how long she had worn glasses, I determined that she had eye problems that necessitated getting glasses during her adolescent years.

We discussed doing Netra Basti as a way of helping her vision and eye strain. Having done this technique with others, I had learned that sometimes a person's eyes go bad at an early age due to emotional trauma—signifying the wish to avoid the sight of unpleasant aspects of life. I was aware from our initial interview that Joyce was an incest survivor. It was, therefore, more than likely that her vision problems were connected to her experiences of incest as a young girl. Joyce elected to try Netra Basti as a means of helping her move forward more quickly in resolving the incest issue that she was dealing with in her counseling sessions.

Joyce experienced the usual reported benefits of Netra Basti during the first two treatments. Dirt imbedded in her eye tissues surfaced in the ghee, leaving her eyes feeling cleaner. Her peripheral vision improved, and her general vision became sharper. It was not until the third treatment, however, that we touched upon visual memories from her past.

Netra Basti is an extremely nurturing treatment, and its comforting qualities allow even the most painful of visual memories to surface without causing catharsis or retraumatization — something that can occur in counseling, where issues may be accelerated faster than psychological integration is possible. In Joyce's case, the visual memories that arose during a deeply relaxing moment came almost as an "ah-hah" experience—a dawning of realization.

From a psychotherapeutic point of view, although in Western culture incest is considered a violation, the familial bond between fathers and daughters often blurs this aspect. (From a Buddhist psychological perspective, this is blurred further by the fact that the bond between fathers and daughters—as well as mothers and sons—is considered a karmic attraction where sexuality does play a part.) The result is that some women learn to armor themselves psychologically by seeing themselves as "special" in their father's eyes rather than violated, the sexual act being an expression of that "specialness."

This is a useful fiction that sometimes helps children cope with pain and confusion. In Joyce's case, her visual memory presented her with a different scenario. Lying in a relaxed manner while the ghee was on her eyes, from the corner of her right eye—the eye which was weakest—she saw her father in her visual memory. Her father was with the babysitter, and they were going into a bedroom. Although Joyce had tried to rationalize her incest experience at an early age by believing that she was special to her father, this illusion was destroyed by the flashback she saw of her father with the babysitter and the realization that he had sex indiscriminately. Even though all therapeutic attempts to get her in touch with the violence done to her had not been successful, the vision of her father going into the bedroom with the babysitter so enraged her that she had come close to destroying her right eye from the anger. She had wanted to blot out this vision by destroying her own eyesight. With this new insight, Joyce was able to go back into counseling with a new focus that was more appropriate to her experience of those traumatic events.

Although this case history is especially dramatic, I have repeatedly seen Netra Basti used as an effective tool in conjunction with counseling and psychotherapy in cases where painful memories have been repressed over the years. This simple yet effective ancient technique can significantly aid clinical endeavors towards psychological transformation.

SHIRO DHARA

Shiro dhara is a process of pouring a fine stream of warm sesame oil on the central fontanelle (or crown) point, or the point above and between the eyes often called the region of the third eye. In the Indian Ayurvedic tradition, the primary point used is the third eye; in Tibetan Ayurveda it is the crown point.

Shiro dhara is deeply relaxing and is intended to clear excess LUNG from the head region. It is useful for the treatment of tension headaches, scalp sensitivity, and mental overstimulation. Dr. Lobsang Rapgay has called this process "psycho-spiritual" massage[10]—and for good reason.

According to Tibetan medicine and Buddhist practice, there is a central spiritual energy channel running through the body. Alongside this spiritual energy channel and crossing over and binding its energy are two smaller channels that start at the tip of the nostrils and end below the navel. Where these *nadis*, namely *roma* and *changma* in Tibetan, cross over and constrict the central channel are the locations of the chakras. In spiritual practice, the intention is to loosen the constriction of these channels and allow the spiritual force of the body to move more freely. The result is a higher level of spiritual integration and awareness as well as *siddhis* (Tibetan, *ngo drup*), or powers such as clairvoyance or the ability to levitate and fly.

By pouring a steady warm stream of sesame oil for a period of twenty to thirty minutes on the third eye, the pressure of the channels around the central channel in this region is diminished. The result is a quieting of the mind, the elimination of discursiveness, and an opening up to greater spiritual energy. It is for these reasons that Shiro dhara is done as preparation for intensive meditation practice and/or retreat. I have observed that the deeply relaxing aspect of Shiro dhara elevates alpha and theta brain wave activity. In such a mental state, answers to profound and perplexing questions arise almost spontaneously. And visions can arise that are useful for those engaged in vision quests. Implicit in these claims and observations is that the person receiving this therapy is mentally and spiritually prepared to be opened up to this degree. Thus, those utilizing this technique need to establish a relationship of trust with the client and have a clear sense of the appropriateness of Shiro dhara.

The following description of Shiro dhara emphasizes the third eye point. This is effective from both the Indian and Tibetan point of view, creating similar results.

In order to do Shiro dhara one needs:

1. one quart of sesame oil
2. a Shiro dhara pot from India or a separatory funnel with ring and stand from a chemical supply shop or chemistry lab
3. a basin in which to catch the oil

The procedure

Have the client lie face up on a massage table or surface that is off the ground. If the person has not already had preliminary Len Nga massage and steam, massage the abdomen and then the head and the head marma points. Place a rolled towel under the neck so that the forehead is tilted back. You want to have the client positioned on the table or surface so that when the oil hits the third eye region, it pours back over the scalp and drains into a bowl beneath the table. Make sure that the person is warm and comfortable and can remain in this position for about thirty minutes.

Warm the sesame oil to just above body temperature and pour it into the Shiro dhara pot or separatory funnel. Place this in the ring on the stand and position the entire apparatus just behind the person's head so that the end of the funnel is about six inches above the forehead region. Turn the stop cock slowly to be sure that the stream is hitting a point just

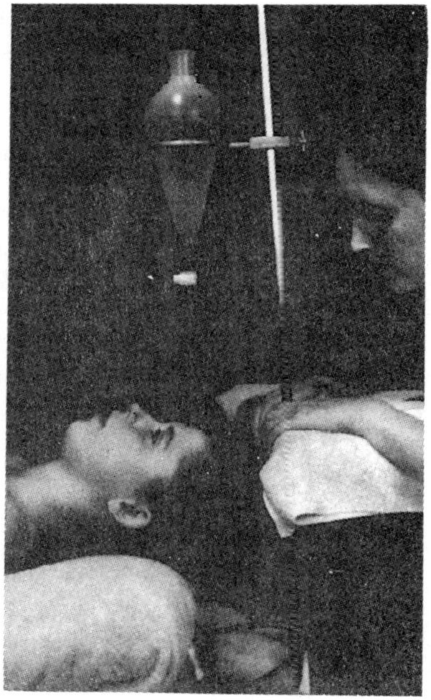

Shiro dhara process.

above and between the eyes but does not drain into the eye sockets. (You may need to adjust the head tilt as well.)

During the time the stream is pouring onto the client's third eye region, remain present and focused. Encourage the client to relax. Soft, contemplative music is useful. You may suggest a focus (a vision, mantra, or problem), but tell the client that he or she should only focus in this way if it is not a strain. As the client lies there, the head may move spontaneously. Also, the forehead angle will change as that region of the face relaxes more. Thus you may need to reposition the stream of oil to ensure that it stays on its mark.

At the end of the Shiro dhara session, encourage the client to move slowly. Since a client is very psychologically impressionable at this time he or she should be encouraged to avoid any stressful situations during the day. (One may wish to talk about the client's schedule prior to the session.) A client should be encouraged to take time to savor the process and should also be told that their sleep for that night and possibly a few subsequent nights may be altered. (Many people report that when they have laid down to sleep, their eyes still feel open.)

In the context of Len Nga therapy, Shiro dhara is done after the steaming process but before the flour cleansing. It can be done on consecutive days towards the latter part of the Len Nga process. At the same time, like other techniques described, it can be used on a onetime basis or out of the context of the Len Nga process, providing the person giving the therapy considers it appropriate. Generally, like all of the Len Nga therapies, a person receiving Shiro dhara should be living a fairly sane and stable lifestyle. It is also advised that the therapist ensure that the client is drug free—of both prescribed and illicit drugs—although Shiro dhara can be useful in the latter stages of recovery from chemical dependency. Shiro dhara seems to be useful in helping to renormalize brain activity and reduce cravings, even though this is only an empirical observation which demands more scientific scrutiny.

TAILORING A GENERAL LEN NGA THERAPY REGIMEN FOR YOU

In the Indian approach to Len Nga therapy, the emphasis is placed on the *kriya*, or cleansing aspect. As a result, the order and intensity of the techniques applied during therapy will differ from the Tibetan approach, where cleansing has its rightful place but is considered a precursor to more important psycho-spiritual transformation.

As a result of the strong cleansing emphasis, Indian Ayurveda takes people through cathartic processes more than Tibetan Ayurveda. Tibetans are concerned that too rapid a physical purification will lead to an increase of LUNG. Thus a person may be having a "far out" experience but may not accomplish the psycho-spiritual integration that is desired from the Len Nga process as taught in the tantras.

This does not mean that Tibetan Len Nga therapy is merely a psycho-spiritual process. Indeed, acute, chronic, and degenerative physical problems can be greatly improved if not altogether eliminated through Len Nga therapy. When there is a lot of physical pain or suffering, it is very difficult to focus on loftier goals. Thus, a Len Nga therapist may actively address physical distress but will never lose sight of the psycho-spiritual dimensions of the person's physical suffering. For in all physical illnesses there will be a psychological and spiritual aspect. Thus the pace taken in therapy is designed to facilitate physical relief, awareness of how such a condition has arisen, and insight into how to proceed in the future. Len Nga therapy should guide one back to one's original rang-zhin so that one's lifestyle and spiritual process are more streamlined and efficiently focused. The case history at the end of the chapter demonstrates how the physical, psychological, and spiritual aspects of one's life can be affected by Len Nga therapy.

This having been said, Tibetans see value in using Len Nga therapy for yearly cleans-ing and renewal. Like Ayurveda in general, yearly cleansing is considered an important dimension of preventive health care. In accordance with the nyepa dominance of one's rang-zhin, a yearly "spring cleaning" can be done as a way of cleansing and retuning one's health for the year. The following chart gives an indication of what each constitutional type can do on a yearly basis for sound preventive health-care maintenance. Single-nyepa constitutions are indicated here. If you are a double-nyepa type, consider what your symptoms are at the time to determine which of the seasonal cleansing times is best for you. It can even be that doing Len Nga at both times is a sound idea. The duration of the Len Nga therapy recommended for these purposes is three to five days.

CLEANSING ACCORDING TO CONSTITUTIONAL TYPE

NYEPA	LUNG	TrIPA	BEKAN
Season	SUMMER SOLSTICE	AUTUMNAL EQUINOX	VERNAL EQUINOX
Massage Technique	oil massage (most oil)	light massage (minimal oil)	salt glow or grainy lotions
	acupressure	acupressure	acupressure
Type of Oil	sesame, juniper, pine, or aquilaria oil	red sandalwood, sesame/ almond mix or sunflower oil	almond, eucalyptus, or ginger oil
Type of Flour	chickpea flour (strong LUNG—use barley flour)	chickpea flour	chickpea flour
Hydrotherapy	warming herbs (ginger, bay, eucalyptus)	cooling, relaxing (barberry, senna, bay, eucalyptus)	invigorating (ginger, licorice, bay, eucalyptus)
Specific Len Nga Techniques	enemas, Na Jong (using ghee)	purgatives and blood washes (using myrobalan or terminalia chebulic)	emetics, Na Jong (using ginger or gor calamus)

Consult an Indian or Tibetan Ayurvedic health-care practitioner familiar with Pancha Karma or Len Nga therapy for more details (see Resources).

REJUVENATION

In the Third Karmapa's treatise entitled "The Profound Inner Meaning," it is explained that when we are born we possess a psychic network of vital channels, nerves, and winds that provide us with the potential for realizing total enlightenment and being able to act in the world effectively.[11] As we age, even if we do not engage in harmful activity, this psychic network deteriorates. If we add to this an imbalanced lifestyle comprised of improper food, a lack of exercise, sexual impropriety, lack of spiritual focus in an unbalanced environment with a host of distractions, it is no wonder that the miraculous stories of men and women who lived well past a century seem like biblical stories, myths, or fairy tales. In our time we are surrounded by chronic and degenerative disease at earlier ages and a life expectancy which has begun to decline.

By living more in tune with our rang-zhin, following good dietary practices, engaging in appropriate exercise, behaving in a way that is balanced and with intention, rather than whimsical, we indeed slow down the aging process. Len Nga therapy can help us to clear out obstructions that arise from not understanding our rang-zhin and to cope with our ever-changing environment. By engaging in spiritual practice, we overcome our mental fixations that keep us out of touch with ourselves, others, and our environment and help us to tap into the powers inherent in the psychic network. It is even said that spiritual practice alone will prolong life since we eliminate the actual cause of negativity.

Tibetans have investigated the aging process and come up with ways to not only slow it down but reverse the process. In his discussion of rejuvenation and virilification, Dr. Yeshe Donden cites examples of teachers of the past who practiced certain meditations and used specific medicines to regain youthfulness.[12] Dr. Donden explains how virilification has both a mundane and spiritual side. In a feudal-based society as Tibet has been, the importance of bloodlines and family lineage are important, and virilification techniques would be used to either have more children or to ensure the begetting of a son as heir so that family wealth and power would be passed on to the next generation. From a more spiritual perspective, the revitalizing of sexual potency is intended to give the spiritual practitioner a greater ability to experience union and bliss in meditative practice, whether it be with or without a sexual partner. As mentioned in our discussion of Len Nga therapy, beyond mundane virilification, rejuvenation serves its purest purpose in restoring body and mind energy for further spiritual transformation.

Consequently, the tantras possess formulas for *Chulen* (Sanskrit: *rasayanas*), or essence extracts, the purpose of which are rejuvenation. Some of them are mere combinations of food sources. Other Chulen are herbs, basmas, and other substances that are painstakingly prepared and taken in ritual fashion. A general prerequisite for the use of such substances is detoxification of the body to aid effectiveness. Thus one cannot bypass sound lifestyle practices and behaviors to go to the fountain of youth.

Regarding the power of such medicines, the following anecdote may be of interest. In 1989, I had an opportunity to spend time with a Western *repa*, or yogi. This yogi, called Rinchen Repa, had lived in Nepal for years. Under the guidance of one of his teachers, he went into solitary retreat in a mountain cave, where he did intensive meditative practice and sustained his body energy solely with a flower essence Chulen. When taken during a retreat or in appropriate ritual fashion, such a Chulen facilitates balanced body functioning, allowing for the harmonious utilization of the LUNG energy of the body, which is most useful in intense meditative practice.

After completing this three-month retreat, Rinchen Repa headed back to Kathmandu. En route he stopped at a local village tea shop. Having had a cup of tea, he was about to leave when he swooned and passed out.

Three days later, Rinchen Repa woke up in the clinic of a local Tibetan doctor. He was informed that he had been poisoned. (In this region of Nepal, lineages of black magic practitioners try to steal the spiritual powers of yogis and teachers by poisoning them. Many lamas have died there as a result.) Further, he was told that the amount of poison he had been given was so large that he should have died instantly. Since he had not, the doctor inquired about Rinchen Repa's prior activities. Upon learning of the Chulen retreat, the doctor said that it was the power of the Chulen that had saved him.

To date, one may learn of different Chulens from Tibetan physicians. Dr. Lobsang Rapgay, for example, prescribes the Chulen 28 formula where appropriate (see Resources). Some of his Western students are researching the other Chulens described in the tantras. As they become tested for their benefits, information about them will be published. Some are general enough that they will no doubt reach the marketplace. Others are only appropriate in spiritual retreats where rejuvenation is the focus.

A LEN NGA THERAPY CASE HISTORY

Joan came to me after she had seen her husband go through a general Len Nga program. Bill's sinus drainage had disappeared along with his hemorrhoids, pelvic tension, and chronic pain from a ten-year-old injury to his shoulder.

Joan's situation was different, however. The mood swings and periodic suicidal thoughts that she had been addressing through psychotherapy had become more unbearable. For further assistance she went to a psychiatrist, who diagnosed manic-depression. The therapy recommended was lithium.

However, two weeks of taking lithium had convinced her that she did not want to be on it. She had always been supersensitive to drugs and medications and thus suffered almost every classic side effect of the lithium, including sweating of the feet and hands and a continuous low-grade nausea. Her first decision was to stop taking the lithium and all prescribed antidepressants. She then proceeded to follow the example of her husband by quitting smoking, cutting her intake of coffee, and eliminating most dairy foods, red meats, and heavy spices for a trial period of one month. Following that she began to see me for periodic Tibetan-style shiatsu sessions. After six weeks of this regimen, she began to improve, but there were still times when her mood swings went beyond a comfortable level. These mood swings would undermine her confidence and sabotage the reasons she had for trying to improve her diet and curb her nicotine and caffeine intake. It was at this point that I spoke with her about doing a Len Nga therapy program to which she agreed.

First, we talked about her general lifestyle. From this I learned of her erratic eating, irregular hours, and resultant bouts with constipation, bloating, gas, and insomnia which when bad enough exacerbated her despair and led to violent outbursts. Interestingly enough on both a cognitive and emotional level she demonstrated a high level of self-understanding; yet it was still not having much impact on her day-to-day functioning. If anything, the dissonance between her awareness and psycho-physical problems was an added source of frustration.

Initially I recommended five days of Len Nga therapy, which we later extended to a week. Three days prior to beginning the treatments I had her start a cleansing diet of basmati rice and spilt mung beans with spices (called kichadi), cooked vegetables, and hot water. In the evening she took a standard Ayurvedic bowel detoxifier.

Daily treatments included herbal steam baths and hot sesame oil massages. Added to this at various points were *nasya*, or nasal administration, herbal enemas, and Shiro dhara.

Days one and two were uneventful, although Joan reported that she was sleeping better and didn't feel bloated. But by day three something happened. Joan came into the session extremely agitated. She expressed feeling a lot of tension, mostly focused in her head, with many racing thoughts. It was almost unbearable for her to lie down to receive a massage. As usual I started with massage of the head. On this occasion I decided to follow this with a ginger-based nasya and then calamus oil.

The results of this procedure were dramatic. Although ginger nasal administration usually stings at first, that effect was short lived in Joan's case. But more noticeable was the tremendous sigh of relief she made. The excess LUNG—the source of the tension and racing thoughts—was being driven from her head. She reported a clarity that she hadn't experienced for years, coupled with deep relaxation. To help this process I applied sustained heat to the abdomen and recommended that she do an herbal enema in the evening.

By the morning of the fourth day, Joan was a changed person, relaxed and light. That feeling continued through the remainder of the seven days. With years of toxicity leaving her system and her body balanced, she was discovering that she had actually made considerable progress in psychotherapy. It was as if her body was finally catching up with her mind. There was a greater sense of integration than she had previously experienced.

Seeing her agitation leave and knowing that she was quite intuitive and wanted to go further in the integrative process, I did Shiro dhara for three consecutive days, the result being a gentle surfacing of images and impressions that were useful in meditations and psychotherapy.

My observation was that Joan was dramatically improved from the Len Nga therapeutic process. This seemed to also be born out in events that followed in Joan's life. Seeing the benefits of massage, subsequently Joan completed a six-month massage training program. Her usual behavior under stress during exams had been to forget about good eating habits, smoke, and drink coffee to stay awake. But now, starting from a more balanced and relaxed state of being, Joan was able to go through the massage program, maintain a regular and supportive lifestyle, and face exams with more clarity than she had previously experienced in similar situations. In addition, many of the other problems she and her husband were facing resolved almost by magic. Shortly thereafter, they moved and Joan started what is now a successful therapeutic massage business.

In the field of mental health counseling, too often lifestyles and body energetic conditions go unexamined and pharmaceutical solutions are provided, the result being the masking of symptoms and the prolongation of suffering. Even though the problem may seem to be more manageable as symptomatic relief is offered, without deeper levels of psychological and somatic experience being addressed, gradual physical and/or mental deterioration is more than likely. Even if clients have a high degree of cognitive awareness of what is going on, the dissonance in their mind-body experience may create a further loss of self-esteem and confidence as they—and the therapist—try to determine why some days they feel good and other days just as bad as before.

As discussed previously, the first level of Tibetan medicine includes the examination of lifestyle, including dietary habits. As we are not accustomed to looking at our day-to-day lives and seeing how habits exacerbate our mental and/or physical state of being, the recommendation to change such habits may seem logical but not necessarily realistic. Adding Len Nga therapy to standard psychological and psychotherapeutic regimens can change this. As the process rebalances us, bringing us closer to our rang-zhin, or original blueprint, we feel nurtured, supported, and stronger on many levels. The result can be a greater confidence in making and sticking to lifestyle changes.

The treatments of detoxification and rejuvenation discussed in this chapter can provide new tools for those whose mental problems are caused by stress. For those whose problems are more deeply seated, they can provide a new gentleness of being that will facilitate more positive and productive resolution.

chapter seven

TIME AND PLACE

This book has presented an extensive amount of information about how we can improve the quality of our lives using the preventive health-care practices of Tibetan Ayurveda and related healing arts. Whether or not such changes will be effective depends on many factors.

The most crucial factor in successfully making changes is the resolve to do so. Without motivation and personal investment, successful change with positive results will elude us. When we feel coerced into changing, we sabotage our efforts.

Along with motivation, we need to have confidence in the methods based on knowledge about them. Because a change of lifestyle not only affects us but also our relationship to others, we should expect challenges to what we are doing. In addition to strong motivation and confidence in the methods, we must have confidence in ourselves. We need to remind ourselves that we are changing to make ourselves stronger, more vital, and better equipped to handle our own lives.

There are three additional factors that need to be addressed when it comes to making successful changes. These have to do with the actual circumstances we find ourselves in when we decide to make changes. Tibetan medicine and tradition offer information on how we can best maximize the use of our circumstances by looking at setting (the place in which we are making the change), and timing (when we plan to make various changes). Lastly, I would like to address the issue of the supportive network around us. Our physical and social environments must be looked at.

In terms of setting and timing, we are talking about becoming familiar with the energetic forces of nature around us. We are made up of the five transformations, or elements, that are identified in Oriental medicine, philosophy, and religion. These elements are not only the building blocks of our psycho-physical existence. They are also the dynamic forces of our environment: the quality of air, the climate, the layout of the land around us, the seasons, and the energy present in the larger cycles of time. There is a continuous dance that we are engaged in where our body with its own set rhythms interacts with elements of the natural environment in which we exist. In their study of nature, the sages of ancient times studied this interaction—this dance—looking for patterns, rhythms, and cycles and how they influenced our bodies, attitudes, and spiritual development. They noted that certain environments and places, times of day, seasons, and larger cycles of time affect us in predictable ways. This is the basis for the use of geomancy and astrology in health-care matters.

SETTING AND GEOMANCY

In Ayurveda, it is said that certain environments will aggravate the nyepas. For example, cold, high, and dry climates will aggravate the nyepa of LUNG. Thus for those with LUNG dominant rang-zhin, such a climate will produce more LUNG symptoms. In such an environment, a LUNG-type person needs to be proactive in health-care maintenance because it is so easy to get out of balance. While hot and humid climates aggravate the nyepa of TRIPA, cold and clammy/damp climates aggravate BEKAN. Thus people with these constitution types need to be mindful in such climates, lest their respective symptoms become more pronounced and problematic.

Although there are climates generally like the ones described above, these climates can be a part of seasonal variation. Thus, given the climate and a person's rang-zhin, there may be one or two seasons in the year during which they need to be a little more cautious and proactive in health-care maintenance. For example, winter in New Mexico is cold, high, and dry—very aggravating for LUNG. Thus, LUNG-type people who live in New Mexico need to stay more focused with LUNG-reducing practices during the winter than in summer. An awareness of your rang-zhin and the nyepa-aggravating or enhancing qualities of your region can help you to stay healthy and balanced throughout the year.

Another important consideration is habitat and home setting. Environmental health at work and home is recognized increasingly as a major health-care issue. The concerns addressed by environmental health-care workers are crowding, pollution, building materials, and so forth. These are not discussed here. However, they are a grosser level of reality that can be understood in the context of the science called geomancy. In Chinese this science is called *feng-shui* and in Tibetan *sache* (pronounced sah-chay). Translated, sache means "earth observation."

The Venerable Tai Situ, Rinpoche, says in his book *Relative World, Ultimate Mind:*

> Of the many possible ways to fulfill the physical and psychological requirements of life—such as comfort and convenience, clarity, tranquillity, and confidence—one important way is to adjust our surroundings. The art of geomancy helps us to do this by removing environmental circumstances that hinder peace of mind and body and creating those that are conducive to it.[1]

Sache can be as general as understanding our position in the universe and in a nation on the planet and the resulting dominant elements present there; or it can be as specific as determining the local forces that influence where best to build a house or where a given room in a house should be. Some rules of sache apply equally to all people regardless of constitution or elemental dominance; others are more specific, where aspects of a person's astrological chart determine beneficial direction, habitat, and so forth.

Situ Rinpoche encourages people to make choices of environment and dwelling based on an understanding of the energetics of the elements:

> The location of your house can affect your health, emotions, personality, finances, and family relations either beneficially or adversely, depending upon whether the surroundings are harmonious or discordant in terms of energy flow.[2]

From this standpoint it is interesting to consider why, for example, certain parts of a city seem more congested, have more crime, or are more polluted. From a limited, everyday point of view it can be easy to blame such conditions on race, socioeconomic factors, or political maneuvers. But is it possible that such places exist because the energies and the ways in which people have established themselves there are not in harmony? We may know of city streets where, within a few blocks of areas where there is turmoil, even with the same racial or socioeconomic mix, people are happy and the streets are orderly. Instead of assuming that problems or success of a given area and people are the result of motivation or mitigating, intractible social and political forces, it may be useful to look at the energetics of an area on the basis of the principles of geomancy.

Regarding health, the literature of geomancy cites examples of people who had some incurable disease and were "miraculously" cured when their bed was moved to another room in the house. In other cases mentioned, families with much inner conflict became harmonious and their financial matters improved when the rooms in their houses were rearranged and the color schemes altered. The book *Feng Shui: The Chinese Art of Placement* by Sarah Rossbach gives numerous testimonials of people's physiological, psychological, and social situations improving after consulting those knowledgeable in this art.[3]

Although a lengthy discussion of geomancy is beyond the scope of this book, readers are encouraged to take environmental factors into account when establishing a viable lifestyle for personal growth.

TIMING AND ASTROLOGY

Throughout this book we have looked at the importance of timing when it comes to engaging in various activities. Some seasonal behaviors apply to all constitutions and some are more constitution-specific. As discussed in the chapter "Nutritional Practices," not only should different types of foods be consumed in different seasons, but people with various constitutions should eat their main meals at different times of the day. Detoxification procedures in Len Nga therapy are not only constitution-specific but should be used during the most efficacious season for cleansing the specific nyepas. Beyond these guidelines, Tibetan astrology, or *kar-tse* (pronounced car-tsay), provides additional information for making such lifestyle practices more effective.

Tibetan astrology is as complex as occidental astrology. It is considered one of the eight worldly sciences that, according to Tai Situ, Rinpoche, "utilize the elements and laws of nature to explain circumstances of life so that one can find the best way to adapt to these circumstances and derive benefit from them."[4] Since we are made up of the elements of nature, we are like a microcosm of the greater cosmos. Tibetans do not consider astrology to be a spiritual practice but rather a worldly one. It can help to create a context in which we most beneficently interact with our world. When we are focused on doing what is most beneficial in the most efficient manner, not only do we become more proficient at what we do, we also experience a greater sense of joy in our constant dance with the universe.

Since 1990 Michael Erlewhine, astrologer and owner of Matrix Software, has published a calendar derived from the Tibetan tradition. The emphasis of this chart is on moon phases and how one can select times of the lunar month most auspicious for doing specific meditational practices. Erlewhine provides an excellent explanation as to how this system works and why it is beneficial in the timing of spiritual endeavors. (To order this calendar, see Resources.)

Even before the publication of these calendars, Erlewhine was at the forefront of introducing Tibetan astrology into the Western arena. In the mid-eighties Matrix sponsored Bhutanese astrologer Sangye Wangchuck to teach rudimentary aspects of Tibetan astrological practice. His main focus was on the mewas, but he also provided some information about the twelve-year cycle of archetypal energy patterns expressed metaphorically as animals. Each animal represents typical personality characteristics of people born in the year of a given animal sign.[5] Derek Walters's *Chinese Astrology* gives a more detailed description of these signs and their implications that is in keeping with the Tibetan tradition. *Tibetan Astrology*, by Phillipe Cornu, has further elucidated these and other intricacies of the Tibetan system.

In the chapter "Meditation and Spiritual Practice" the material as presented by Sangye Wangchuck is incorporated with sources from other cultures that use this system to create narratives that are useful for those engaged in their own spiritual pursuit. These mewas also can provide useful information on general personality traits, health concerns, relationship issues, career choices, travel, and moving. My book *Nine-Star Ki: Your Astrological Companion to Feng Shui* takes the Tibetan material and looks at it in the context of the Nine House astrology of China and the Nine-Star Ki system of Japan, both of which are none other than the mewa system as seen from the perspective of these other cultures (see Bibliography).

The chart below gives you the mewa number and animal sign for specific years. Bear in mind that the Tibetan or Chinese calendar used for the animal sign is based on lunar cycles and sets the beginning of the year—for the most part—toward the end of January through the middle of February. There are other systems within Tibetan astrology that will set the New Year earlier or later. When it comes to the mewas, or what is called the Nine Star Ki, a different calendar is used that sets the beginning of the year almost exactly at February 4, the date that is equidistant from the winter solstice and the vernal equinox.

When reading the chart below, I recommend the following strategy. For selecting your animal sign, rely on the month and date indicated in the "start of year" column. If your birth date falls prior to the date that is set as the first lunar calendar day of that year, select your animal sign from the previous year. For the mewa always use February 4 as the beginning of the year. If your birth date falls between January 1 and February 3, select your mewa from the previous year.

For our purposes, the data provided for each year are the year's mewa, animal, and element. Mewas rotate through the years on a nine-year cycle, elements on a ten-year cycle, with each element appearing in two consecutive years, and animal signs rotate on a twelve-year cycle. Information for the animals and the elements is found below. Mewa information is found in chapter 5 and in appendix 4.

YEAR	START OF YEAR	MEWA#	ELEMENT	ANIMAL
1905	Feb. 8	5	Wood	Snake
1906	Feb. 22	4	Fire	Horse
1907	Feb. 10	3	Fire	Sheep
1908	Mar. 2	2	Earth	Monkey
1909	Feb. 24	1	Earth	Bird
1910	Feb. 12	9	Iron	Dog

YEAR	START OF YEAR	MEWA#	ELEMENT	ANIMAL
1911	Feb. 26	8	Iron	Pig
1912	Feb. 20	7	Water	Mouse
1913	Feb. 7	6	Water	Ox
1914	Feb. 22	5	Wood	Tiger
1915	Feb. 16	4	Wood	Hare
1916	Feb. 4	3	Fire	Dragon
1917	Feb. 24	2	Fire	Snake
1918	Feb. 11	1	Earth	Horse
1919	Mar. 4	9	Earth	Sheep
1920	Feb. 20	8	Iron	Monkey
1921	Feb. 7	7	Iron	Bird
1922	Feb. 28	6	Water	Dog
1923	Feb. 16	5	Water	Pig
1924	Feb. 4	4	Wood	Mouse
1925	Feb. 24	3	Wood	Ox
1926	Feb. 11	2	Fire	Tiger
1927	Mar. 4	1	Fire	Hare
1928	Feb. 22	9	Earth	Dragon
1929	Feb. 10	8	Earth	Snake
1930	Mar. 1	7	Iron	Horse
1931	Feb. 18	6	Iron	Sheep
1932	Feb. 7	5	Water	Monkey
1933	Feb. 25	4	Water	Bird
1934	Feb. 14	3	Wood	Dog
1935	Mar. 5	2	Wood	Pig
1936	Feb. 23	1	Fire	Mouse
1937	Feb. 12	9	Fire	Ox
1938	Mar. 3	8	Earth	Tiger
1939	Feb. 20	7	Earth	Hare
1940	Feb. 9	6	Iron	Dragon
1941	Feb. 27	5	Iron	Snake
1942	Feb. 16	4	Water	Horse
1943	Feb. 5	3	Water	Sheep
1944	Feb. 24	2	Wood	Monkey
1945	Feb. 13	1	Wood	Bird
1946	Mar. 4	9	Fire	Dog
1947	Feb. 21	8	Fire	Pig
1948	Feb. 10	7	Earth	Mouse
1949	Feb. 28	6	Earth	Ox
1950	Feb. 17	5	Iron	Tiger
1951	Feb. 7	4	Iron	Hare
1952	Feb. 26	3	Water	Dragon

YEAR	START OF YEAR	MEWA#	ELEMENT	ANIMAL
1953	Feb. 14	2	Water	Snake
1954	Mar. 5	1	Wood	Horse
1955	Feb. 23	9	Wood	Sheep
1956	Feb. 12	8	Fire	Monkey
1957	Mar. 2	7	Fire	Bird
1958	Feb. 19	6	Earth	Dog
1959	Feb. 8	5	Earth	Pig
1960	Feb. 27	4	Iron	Mouse
1961	Feb. 16	3	Iron	Ox
1962	Feb. 5	2	Water	Tiger
1963	Feb. 24	1	Water	Hare
1964	Feb. 14	9	Wood	Dragon
1965	Mar. 4	8	Wood	Snake
1966	Feb. 21	7	Fire	Horse
1967	Feb. 10	6	Fire	Sheep
1968	Feb. 29	5	Earth	Monkey
1969	Feb. 17	4	Earth	Bird
1970	Feb. 7	3	Iron	Dog
1971	Feb. 26	2	Iron	Pig
1972	Feb. 15	1	Water	Mouse
1973	Mar. 5	9	Water	Ox
1974	Feb. 23	8	Wood	Tiger
1975	Feb. 12	7	Wood	Hare
1976	Mar. 1	6	Fire	Dragon
1977	Feb. 19	5	Fire	Snake
1978	Feb. 8	4	Earth	Horse
1979	Feb. 27	3	Earth	Sheep
1980	Feb. 17	2	Iron	Monkey
1981	Feb. 5	1	Iron	Bird
1982	Feb. 24	9	Water	Dog
1983	Feb. 13	8	Water	Pig
1984	Mar. 3	7	Wood	Mouse
1985	Feb. 20	6	Wood	Ox
1986	Feb. 9	5	Fire	Tiger
1987	Feb. 28	4	Fire	Hare
1988	Feb. 18	3	Earth	Dragon
1989	Feb. 7	2	Earth	Snake
1990	Feb. 26	1	Iron	Horse
1991	Feb. 15	9	Iron	Sheep
1992	Mar. 5	8	Water	Monkey
1993	Feb. 22	7	Water	Bird
1994	Feb. 11	6	Wood	Dog

YEAR	START OF YEAR	MEWA#	ELEMENT	ANIMAL
1995	Mar. 2	5	Wood	Pig
1996	Feb. 19	4	Fire	Mouse
1997	Feb. 8	3	Fire	Ox
1998	Feb. 27	2	Earth	Tiger
1999	Feb. 17	1	Earth	Hare
2000	Mar. 7	9	Iron	Dragon
2001	Feb. 24	8	Iron	Snake
2002	Feb. 13	7	Water	Horse
2003	Mar. 3	6	Water	Sheep
2004	Feb. 21	5	Wood	Monkey
2005	Feb. 9	4	Wood	Bird
2006	Feb. 28	3	Fire	Dog
2007	Feb. 18	2	Fire	Pig
2008	Feb. 7	1	Earth	Mouse
2009	Feb. 25	9	Earth	Ox
2010	Feb. 14	8	Iron	Tiger
2011	Mar. 5	7	Iron	Hare
2012	Feb. 22	6	Water	Dragon
2013	Feb. 11	5	Water	Snake
2014	Mar. 2	4	Wood	Horse

Please note that there are several traditions in Tibetan astrology for establishing the starting date for the year. The dates listed in this chart come from the Tsurphu tradition.

THE ELEMENTS

Similar to the Western zodiac signs, which are ascribed to people born during certain time periods, Tibetan astrology ascribes to each of us an animal sign and an element based on the year we were born. Animal signs represent archetypal energies present in a given year that accentuate in us certain external characteristics and behaviors. The element of the year is a further influence that fortifies certain traits in our character over time, regardless of the mewa or animal sign. Briefly, in terms of character, the traits each element accentuates are as follows:

WOOD (also known at times as Tree, Space, or Ether)—creativity, impulsiveness, energy that increases (both mentally and physically), and youthfulness

FIRE—energetic, joyful, warm, quick, intense, transformative

EARTH—grounded, solid, stable, consolidating

IRON (also known as Metal or Air)—maturity, confident strength, malleability, decisiveness, reflective

WATER—fluid, enigmatic, gentle, foresight

So that you may become familiar with your animal attributes we offer brief explanations of each animal sign below. Further on in this text, the reader will be able to use knowledge of the animals for two other purposes.

First, in regard to timing, Dr. Lobsang Rapgay has extracted from the Tibetan astrological material useful information on how each animal sign is influenced by particular days of the week.[6] He has identified days of the week that are "favorable," "friendly," and "antagonistic." A "favorable" day is the best day of the week for you—a time to initiate changes, start ventures, undergo medical procedures, or begin preventive health-care measures. A "friendly" day is one complementary to your sign; it is positive to select for events if you are not able to arrange matters on your "favorable" day. Most other days are relatively neutral, except the "antagonistic" day. An "antagonistic" day is one to avoid when planning events or making changes and you should be more mindful of health and personal matters.

WHEN YOUR TIBETAN ZODIAC ANIMAL SIGN IS . . .	YOUR FAVORABLE DAY IS . . .	YOUR FRIENDLY DAY IS . . .	YOUR ANTAGONISTIC DAY IS . . .
Mouse	Wednesday	Tuesday	Saturday
Ox	Saturday	Wednesday	Thursday
Tiger	Thursday	Saturday	Friday
Hare	Thursday	Saturday	Friday
Dragon	Sunday	Wednesday	Thursday
Snake	Tuesday	Friday	Wednesday
Horse	Tuesday	Friday	Wednesday
Sheep	Friday	Monday	Thursday
Monkey	Friday	Thursday	Tuesday
Bird	Friday	Thursday	Tuesday
Dog	Monday	Wednesday	Thursday
Pig	Wednesday	Tuesday	Saturday

The second reason for including information on the animal signs has to do with compatibilities. Although this strays from place and timing as a focus, it serves as a segue into the remainder of the discussion in this chapter.

When the Ganden Shartse monks passed through the midwest on tour, a colleague of mine asked one of the traveling *geshes* (pronounced geh-shay, which is similar to having a Ph.D. in religion) why there was so much illness and suffering at this time. The geshe's response was somewhat simplistic, but profoundly to the point; "Bad food and bad friends," was his response.

So much has been discussed in this volume regarding diet, general lifestyle, and adapting a more mindful, if not spiritual orientation in one's life. And although we have touched upon the issues of ethics and morality in our interactions, nothing specific has been discussed regarding relationships.

The great Tibetan physician-saint Gampopa once said that a sign of a superior person was that he or she treated all with equanimity, yet still had a few good friends. This is in keeping with the Mahayana Buddhist perspective that on the ultimate level, we are all the same—we all have Buddhanature and Buddha potential. On a relative level, however, some are more in touch with this truth than others, hence the wide variety of human expressions—from the most saintly to the most horrific. And, based on our own Three Poisons (ignorance, attachment, and aggression), we see some whom we are attracted to, others whom we want nothing to do with, and still others who come and go in our lives that we have no particular preference for one way or the other. Buddhist masters encourage their students to see everyone on the highest or ultimate level—as Buddhas. If one cannot do this, in the evolutionary process of developing equanimity in our relations there is the humanistic view that one should just be open to dealing with and overcoming whatever poison arises from a relationship that we have cultivated (intentionally or not) in our lives. Indeed, this is ultimately a very noble approach.

At the same time, Tibetans are very pragmatic. Although such an approach is generally true and good, life is short. If we are going to engage someone in business, marriage, or some other serious relationship, why not use whatever data is available to us to create the most optimal (albeit relative) conditions for a suitable and happy outcome?

Here in the West, we see from marriage statistics that choice based on intuition or attraction does not ensure a "happily-ever-after" scenario and "until death do us part" is just a formality that we seem to only briefly commit ourselves to. In the realm of work, the research I did while working on my masters degree indicated that what made work satisfying or stressful was not how much money one was making, but how well one got on with one's fellow workmates. In both the spheres of personal relationships and work/career matters, a wide array of psycho-emotional testing instruments have been devised by psychologists to ensure better outcomes in everything from dating to long-term job placement and satisfaction. Still, the limitations of the impact of these techniques is revealed by persistent high divorce rates and job-related stress.

Somewhere between blind leaps of faith and Western scientific method lies data culled over time from the observation and experience of seers and adepts. This is the basis for the animal archetypes, elements, and mewas as found in the Tibetan astrological tradition. Tibetan astrology teaches that as we interact with people of various signs, we find that we have more harmonious interactions with those whose signs we are compatible with, while interactions fraught with varying levels of confusion or conflict tend to arise with those whose signs are not compatible with ours. Thus, when approaching or entering into a long-term or significant relationship, why not choose a smoother route?

At the same time, does this mean that we should avoid those who have incompatible signs? Sometimes this is useful, but more often than not, impractical. In fact, for whatever reason, we may even find that we are continually attracted to those whose signs we are least compatible with. What should one do then? Here is where not taking oneself too seriously, overcoming dualistic fixation or rigid thinking by finding methods to cut through the Three Poisons, and a good dose of humor come in. In other words, we make the best of it and grow as individuals. Sometimes the only way around is through, the outcome of which may be greater tolerance and compassion.

A brief description of each animal sign follows along with compatibilities. Although they are not too dissimilar from what is recommended in Chinese horoscopes, the Tibetans see the signs that the Chinese consider as most auspicious for marriage and partnership (what I list below as "Friendly") as having some difficulties. After a private conversation with a Tibetan teacher who was knowledgeable about astrology but wanted to speak off the record, it seems that the reason for the reservation with respect to the ones most favored by the Chinese is that these are the people we usually find ourselves attracted to when we are feeling positive and in the right frame of mind for forming a wholesome, loving relationship. As many astrologers were monks with vows of celibacy, these would obviously be the people they would want to stay away from.

MOUSE: You are charming and enjoy the company of others. Although sociable, your refined and quiet nature creates around you only a small circle of close, but lasting friendships. People can rely on you, but often don't acknowledge your efforts on their behalf. What may be the cause for this is that while amiable and calm on the surface, you can be somewhat manipulative and aggressive. This can create mixed feelings and impressions about you. Ambitious and with a tendency toward self-centeredness, you can be quite calculating. You do think well on your feet and have a strong discerning mind. You have a keen appreciation for wealth and love to collect things around you for the sheer pleasure of doing so. Yet, you may likewise find yourself spending and giving away what is yours heedlessly. Although greater opportunities may pass your way, you prefer to set your sights on more modest goals to ensure success.

Least Compatible with Horse. Not Very Compatible with Hare or Bird. Friendly with Dragon and Monkey. Most Compatible with all other signs.

OX: You have a strength that allows you to feel secure in yourself. You can handle whatever comes your way in your own characteristically slow and methodical way. You don't like to be pushed or prompted. It only annoys you when people try to prompt or compete with you. If people want to change your mind, they need to appeal to your sense of logic. Such a way of being shows patience, but often leads others to see you as unambitious. Still, they appreciate your good nature and dependability. You are very accepting of others as they are, and expect them to be the same of you. This leads you to generally be faithful in relationships. But, if you are betrayed, your almost naive nature can turn to more underhanded methods.

Least Compatible with Sheep. Not Very Compatible with Dragon or Dog. Friendly with Bird and Snake. Most Compatible with all other signs.

TIGER: You are both bold and proud and draw people to you with your charisma. You may appear rash and rough in your behavior, as you like being candid. You seem unrestrained and larger than life. You love competition and have disdain for hierarchy. Convention easily bores you. Such boldness and the aura you project, however, can blind others to your sensitivity and an underlying meekness. When pushed you may conceal your vulnerability with a hot temper. You love taking chances and usually succeed in what you do. You are strongly devoted to those you cherish, but can have difficulties being faithful.

Least Compatible with Monkey. Not Very Compatible with Snake or Pig. Friendly with Horse and Dog. Most Compatible with all other signs.

HARE: Your life seems charmed and full of opportunity. This is mainly because of the fact that you tend to primarily look out for your own interests. You appreciate the aesthetic and your natural articulateness gives you an air of sophistication. Always wanting peace, you abhor conflicts. Thus you can be an excellent diplomat, being charming even to your enemies. However, if pushed you can be devious in your actions and may use gossip as one of your weapons. You would prefer to avoid such situations as you are more cunning than brave. You may appear self-contained and smug. Yet, you are affectionate and shy.

Least Compatible with Bird. Not Very Compatible with Horse or Mouse. Friendly with Sheep and Pig. Most Compatible with all other signs.

DRAGON: You are elegant in appearance, which allows your decisive ways to carry more weight than they actually have. Your "bark is bigger than your bite," even though some may recoil at your short temper. However, you never mean harm. You are just rather grand and dramatic. This coupled with your fascination for life's mysteries leads you to have a life that is vital, yet complex. You do not like to overextend yourself, but will always do what you are called upon to do. Once called upon, you seldom give up until you are victorious—even if the costs are high. You have a hard time containing yourself and can be overly talkative with a tendency to cherish your opinion over the wisdom of others; yet you are an excellent listener and are noted for your sincerity. You can be demanding of others, yet will easily forgive. Your health is better than most, but if you get sick, it can be serious.

Least Compatible with Dog. Not Very Compatible with Sheep or Ox. Friendly with Mouse and Monkey. Most Compatible with all other signs.

SNAKE: You possess a wisdom that comes from having a good sense of what the future holds. Your optimism in how you see things is based on having strong views, a stubborn streak, and the personal sense that no one can really get in your way. You always intend to do what is right, but you are somewhat naive. If challenged too directly, your demeanor can become rough and your temper violent. This can make you the target for rumors and scandals. These can bother you deeply as you can be quite concerned with how others see you as well as how you see yourself. Be aware that your tendencies toward jealousy and possessiveness are the root of many of the difficulties you face. Enjoy your sensual nature, but avoid obsession.

Least Compatible with Pig. Not Very Compatible with Monkey or Tiger. Friendly with Ox and Bird. Most Compatible with all other signs.

HORSE: You have a rather paradoxical nature, which leads you to have many ups and downs in life. Generally you are athletic, fond of adventure, and popular and attractive to the opposite sex. This can create for you a very busy social life. You may act independent, but the truth is that you need people; you need to be valued. This may account for your seeming intolerance and impatience for others when recognition is not forthcoming. Yet, when people acknowledge you and give you the space you need, you have almost miraculous powers and can exert great effort. This is especially true when you are focusing on helping others. Possibly because age has a tempering effect, Horses often find that the second half of life is easier than the first. Beware of your impatience. It can lead to precipitous action with disastrous results.

Least Compatible with Mouse. Not Very Compatible with Bird or Hare. Friendly with Tiger and Dog. Most Compatible with all other signs.

SHEEP: Like the thick wool of a sheep, your exterior conceals much of what happens under the surface. You have original ideas, but they are disguised by your conservative air and fastidious nature that makes you very economical with words. You don't like to make a show of yourself, thus you'll work in the background, taking your time, trying to get things done in accordance with methods that you might not have thought through. Yet, there's no harm in this. You are good natured and good tempered and though you may be a bit gruff, people sense in you a person making efforts on their behalf. You make an exemplary team player. You worry too much, which may be the reason why you can sometimes find yourself overeating. You feel best with a partner with whom you feel protected.

Least Compatible with Ox. Not Very Compatible with Dog or Dragon. Friendly with Pig and Hare. Most Compatible with all other signs.

MONKEY: You are intelligent, inventive, and show a lot of enthusiasm, with many grand ideas. Being very talkative to the point of seeming hyperactive, you can be quite convincing with your plans and schemes. Yet beneath this rather bold exterior and the praise you bestow upon yourself, you are really quite insecure and can crumble easily if you are not taken seriously or are questioned too deeply. This can be the cause of your seeming bad temper, which is nothing more than a ruse to conceal the confusion you are experiencing. Still, you are agile and easily figure out what's going on. "Whatever it takes" is a good personal motto. It probably works to your advantage to be as playful as you are. In love you bear the passion and seductiveness of an adolescent.

Least Compatible with Tiger. Not Very Compatible with Pig or Snake. Friendly with Dragon and Mouse. Most Compatible with all other signs.

BIRD: Like the cock that crows precisely at dawn, you have an alert, precise mind that allows you to catch wind of what is going on ahead of the others. This gives you an air of eccentricity, which you embellish with your flair for extravagance in dress and personal effect. Friends enjoy being with you, as you are interesting and knowledgeable and at the same time streetwise. Thus your manner can be frank, sometimes abrasive. Your advice to friends is helpful, but your tendency toward self-centeredness can make you ignore for yourself the wisdom you offer to others. Still, if you fail in an endeavor, there's always the next time. You have a strong sexual nature and you probably express your most competitive tendencies in your pursuit of love and relationships. You are most hurt by being ignored.

Least Compatible with Hare. Not Very Compatible with Mouse or Horse. Friendly with Ox and Snake. Most Compatible with all other signs.

DOG: How you are viewed depends on whom you are viewed by. Some see you as self-centered and somewhat mean. Perhaps your constant mental activity and need to move about makes them uncertain of your intentions and your relationship with them. There are those, on the other hand, who find you sociable, reliable, and honest. To these people you show a tenacious loyalty and are generous with your time and efforts, exhibiting a willingness to defend them against any form of abusive talk or action. Your pride is not so much in yourself, but in having relationships with people you honor and respect. Some will always be suspicious of your actions and intentions, while others will always give you the benefit of the doubt. You are both vital and virile by nature; a lust for life that is difficult to satisfy and at times, gets in the way of your accomplishing what you want. The cause of this may be your keen analytical mind, which often leads you to take life too seriously. Pessimism and lost opportunity can be the result.

Least Compatible with Dragon. Not Very Compatible with Ox or Sheep. Friendly with Horse and Tiger. Most Compatible with all other signs.

PIG: You are not an original thinker but can accomplish much through your industrious and practical approach to what you want. What you want, however, is rather vague. Thus while you can easily acquire anything, you can end up with a very mixed bag; some good, some bad, some useful, some useless. This seeming lack of discrimination may arise more out of your somewhat naive, easygoing nature and preference for not speaking up, than out of poor judgment. Regardless, you are generally content with the sum total of what comes your way. This basic sense of contentment can give you a noble air. But, such nobility is very dependent on the company you keep. In the presence of people with positive, uplifting ways, you can be the most positive and uplifting. In the presence of lowlifes, you can be the lowest of the low. Regardless of the lifestyle you chose, there is discipline in it. The friends you make are usually lifelong, and you enjoy home life. This does not mean that you are domestic, however. You are more than willing to help out. It's just that if the house is messy, that's OK; if the house is clean, that's OK too. This can be trying to a discriminating spouse or partner and such a laissez-faire approach can be the cause of marital strife. Still, your natural chivalry makes your partner and family feel that you care, even though your mannerisms around affection, and emotions in general, may be rough around the edges.

Least Compatible with Snake. Not Very Compatible with Tiger or Monkey. Friendly with Sheep and Hare. Most Compatible with all other signs.

AMBIENCE AND SOCIAL SUPPORT

When you make a decision to change your lifestyle, it not only impacts you physically, emotionally, and spiritually, but also has an impact on everyone you come into contact with.

Say, for example, you change what, when, and how you eat. You were going out in the evening for late night pizza with your friends a few nights a week. Becoming aware of your rang-zhin and a desire to feel better, you start to focus on eating earlier in the day and not indulging in late night snacks. Suddenly you change the dynamics between yourself and your friends. Perhaps after work you would "unwind" by going to a cocktail lounge for a couple of drinks. Now, you go home to do some exercise and meditation, eliminating time you would have normally spent with friends. The result may be that your friends feel that you are more distant, or even disapproving of what they do. They may think that something is wrong, that you've become a health nut, a hypochondriac, or a fanatic of some sort. Similarly, if you cook for a household and you become sensitive to your own rang-zhin and those of your family members, food preparation may become more complicated and time consuming, or they may not like what you fix and object to the changes. Thus, while motivation and confidence are very important when making lifestyle changes, so are *compassion, patience, and the willingness to communicate* with others to avoid misunderstandings and gain the support of friends and family.

With these thoughts in mind, when it comes to making changes in your lifestyle, the following suggestions may be useful.

1. If you have a specific health concern for which you are seeing a health-care professional, discuss with them the changes you wish to make.

2. Create a personal environment that is conducive to orderly change. If someone in your community is knowledgeable about geomancy, seek their guidance in creating the optimal space to effect changes. Utilize the astrological information provided in this book as well or contact one of the source people or organizations listed in the Resources. If you have concerns about your interactions with some people, get astrological data on them as well. This information can be particularly useful when approaching others close to you.

3. When possible, find people in your community who are interested in preventive health-care practices, especially

those discussed in this book. In order to gain insight into our habitual tendencies and how our social environment can reinforce such patterns and act as an impediment to changes, it is useful to share experiences and knowledge with people of like mind to reinforce the changes you wish to make. Read source material listed in the Bibliography and contact various groups or organizations listed in the Resources that have the knowledge to further your studies and changes; this will provide you with a greater network to support you in your efforts. Try to meet competent Tibetan and Indian Ayurvedic practitioners who may come to your area or invite such practitioners to your area for your benefit and the benefit of others. This is also an excellent way to create a supportive local network. When possible, participate in a retreat or seminar with a competent teacher to deepen your knowledge and appreciation of Ayurvedic practices.

4. If people closest to you are interested and supportive, wonderful. If not, try to understand their point of view and be compassionate, patient, and receptive. Reflect on what brought you to the point of wanting to make changes. Remember, your proselytizing will be considered a nuisance at the least and at worst, an affront to the chosen lifestyle of those close to you. As you become more balanced, have more vitality, and begin to embrace more of the world with a deeper spiritual commitment, you will inspire those around you. Your lifestyle and transformation will speak for themselves. Even if this does not inspire lifestyle changes with those around you, the acceptance and kindness you show yourself will inevitably lead you to be more accepting of them, allowing them to travel their own life's journey.

It is my fervent hope that as you live in accordance with your rang-zhin, your original blueprint, that your life will unfold as it was designed. This is the ultimate goal of medical practices of Tibetan Ayurveda and healing.

May your body be like a rainbow.
May your actions be spontaneous and joyful.
May you experience the limitless potentials of your mind.
And, may you benefit all.

appendix one

EGO AND SUFFERING
A BUDDHIST VIEW

Because our ignorance obscures our ability to understand ourselves or the world, we develop erroneous views, and confusion begins to build. We become attached to this way or that way, thinking that by doing this or that, by eating this or that, by being with this person rather than that person, everything will be perfect. Although none of us really wants to suffer, regardless of how suitable circumstances are, because of our limited view, it is likely that we will experience disappointment as things do not work out as planned or hoped. The result is frustration or anger. Then we become more zealous, refusing to acknowledge our errors of judgment or action. We push away what we perceive as standing in the way of our perfect little universe. And we hold on even tighter to what we think we have accomplished, becoming more and more aggressive.

By description, we have defined what in the medical tantras and in Buddhist teaching is called the Three Poisons: attachment, aggression , and ignorance. These three are the binding forces of the ego and cause all our physical, emotional, and spiritual suffering. They are the basis of self-limited reality that needs to be transcended.

Although they are called poisons, they are like unripe fruits. Attachment, aggression, and ignorance, while being the source of all our suffering, represent an immature picture of reality according to the Buddhist tantric view; they contain enlightened potential, like unripe fruits that become ripe, juicy, and edible. Cutting through attachment, aggression, and ignorance is a matter of not buying into the self-limited reality they portray. When we do not get stuck in self-importance, we open up more. According to some teachings, attachment becomes transformed into wisdom, aggression into useful clarity and compassion, ignorance into skillful activity. Because of the belief that such potentials are always within us, though veiled, Buddhism adheres to the notion that we are inherently good. What we need are the means to relate to the poisons properly in order to transform them into positive ways of being. A good friend and lama, Ole Nydahl, once likened this transformation to tempering steel. When you heat up steel, it goes through a stage of oxidizing and getting blackened. If you take the metal out at that stage, you would end up with a mess. But if you leave it in the heat longer, the black falls away and the steel is transformed, becoming bright, shining, and virtually indestructible.

KARMA AND BIRTH

If our true potential is to be as a Buddha, it may seem fair to ask why we are not perfect already. Questions such as this are central to all religions and have often led to heated debate or even warfare. Discussions on such topics as the origin of life, the nature of God, and our relation to the divine are at best interesting and at worst destructive.

As is the case with many of the inscrutable teachings of the East, the question why is not particularly useful. We need to start at a more basic level—with ourselves. If we begin to understand the mechanisms of our own lives, then, as we become more in touch with our potentials, answers to "why" and other cosmic questions no longer remain mere cognitions but become instead living vibrant truths experienced at the most basic levels of our being. Then the separation between ourselves and our world dissolves, and the question "why" is answered by our own existence.

Until that time, we are under the influence of a self-limited reality, defined by the degree to which we are caught up in the Three Poisons of ignorance, attachment, and aggression. From a Tibetan medical point of view, ignorance, attachment, and aggression are the root causes of what appears as our mind, body, and activity respectively. That is, our perception of our minds, our body, and our capabilities is determined by the self-limiting Three Poisons.

We get all romantic about conception, birth, and babies. In

truth, what is really wonderful about the whole process is that it is an indication of the yearning of the spirit for self-actualization or awakening. Our conception has come about due to unresolved feelings of yearning. As our consciousness migrates from death, it is attracted to a new birth situation based on the positive and negative impressions left in our consciousness from our previous existence. This is reincarnation. For more information on reincarnation, see the Bibliography. We are attracted to the energy created between a mating couple (our parents) and their environment; at the same time, however, this is far from being a conscious choice unless one is close to being, or already is, a completely awakened being. True, we make choices in our lives that determine our future karma (a concept which is in keeping with the biblical notion that what you sow so shall you reap), but once we have died we are more or less experiencing the result of our actions. This is the karma for our future life. Factors such as how we have shaped our consciousness, how or whether we have transcended self-limiting views become the impetus that compels us towards that with which it feels in resonance.

The Venerable Tai Situ Rinpoche has taught that the separation between our consciousness and the natural elements that make up our physical being has a force more powerful than the worst imaginable earthquake.[1] Without some level of mastery, we swoon from the force and find ourselves spinning out of our previous life in a trajectory predetermined by our choices and the resultant karma. The environment and parents we end up with are, indeed, of our own making; yet this is not a conscious decision for the majority. Those capable of withstanding the shock of separation between elements and consciousness by virtue of their meditative discipline enter into another sentient form by choice—be it human, animal, or whatever—are conscious incarnates, known in Tibetan as *tulkus*. Such an occurrence is rare, and the knowledge such conscious incarnates bring into a new life is the sum total of their training in previous lives. Thus, they are called "Rinpoches," or precious ones.

The fact that most beings are compelled to be born rather than consciously choosing to do so should not be considered as negative, however, for it is a blessing to be born. Having a body to relate to and sense fields to interact with in the world gives us a new opportunity to overcome self-limitations and reach our full potentials.

In our past lives, each of us has caught glimpses of and even perhaps learned to cut through our ignorance, our attachment, and our aggression to a greater or lesser extent. Generally, not all Three Poisons, therefore, are of equal strength in various individuals. Perhaps we have done better at curbing our aggression than dispelling our ignorance or attachment. Or perhaps we've given up a lot of illusions but still find ourselves fixated and angry. Whatever we have overcome or not overcome represents the type of consciousness that finds itself once again in the world. This consciousness is the source of all our strengths and weaknesses. As such, it is the blueprint for our enlightenment, for it shows us what resources we have and what needs to be worked on in this lifetime.

According to Buddhist tradition, there are eighty-four thousand possible configurations of the Three Poisons in which one or more is dominant to a varying degree. The Buddhist religious teachings which are a part of the fourth level of Tibetan medicine address how these different configurations can be transformed into their true potential. And in the East, since psyche and soma, or mind and body, are seen as a continuum rather than separate from each other, the medical tantras address the physical and behavioral manifestations of the different configurations of consciousness. Like the notion of genetics in Western medical science, Tibetan medicine posits that along with the mix of attachment, aggression, and ignorance that enters into physical manifestation as a baby comes physiological and psychological predispositions that need to be attended to in the course of the person's life cycle. In the West we call this "constitution." The Sanskrit word for constitution is *prakruti.* The Tibetan word is *rang-zhin.*

Although each one of the poisons is a state of mind, since mind and body are inseparable, each one of them colors our perception of what we are in relation to the world around us. They determine what we actually think our three-dimensional body is made of and the psychological style with which we interact with others and the world. The path that leads from the Three Poisons as thought forms to the intention of physiological manifestation in the three-dimensional world follows a predictable pattern, expounded in Buddhist philosophy as the Doctrine of Interdependent Origination, or Twelve *Nidanas.*

The Twelve Nidanas, although a philosophical explanation of how we become born, are also the process we experience moment to moment as we feel, discriminate, and make choices.

Ignorance is considered the fundamental poison we experience, causing a dualistic split between ourselves and the world due to a lack of clear understanding. On one level this lack of understanding is innocent in that it arises from immaturity. However, reinforced over time, it can become an active process whereby we "ignore" the truth that is front of our noses. At this point, our ignorance is tainted with pride. Pride is considered a *klesa,* or mental obscuration.

With ignorance, the clear and unimpeded nature of our mind is not recognized. Some "thing" begins to emerge. According to the tantras, out of a dynamic emptiness which is the actual nature of our mind when fully realized, forms arise. These forms are none other than projections of the mind. This is expressed in the great Heart Sutra:

> O Sariputra, form is emptiness and the very emptiness is form; emptiness does not differ from form, form does not differ from emptiness; whatever is form, that is emptiness, whatever is emptiness that is form, the same is true of feelings, perceptions, impulses and consciousness . . .[2]

This is the foundation upon which the Tibetan medical tantras are based. Although it is an extremely subtle point that takes years of philosophical inquiry and meditation to grasp, there is no greater achievement in human consciousness than realizing this point in awareness and action.

Out of ignorance, the self-limitation that arises creates an identification with what appears in the mind, as if it were separate from the mind itself. This content is the impressions from past karma. Thus begins the formation of what we identify as ourselves and that which we identify as other than ourselves.

From the dualistic distinction between self and other, there arises a sense of "I" that appears as permanent. It is called consciousness, the third nidana (the first two being ignorance and this identification which is called formation, the first dualistic notion). According to the Venerable Khenpo Karthar, Rinpoche, consciousness is the product of previously accumulated karma, the feelings associated with that karma with which we identify, and a spark of intelligence which gives us the potential to unravel our fixations in the future if we so choose.[3] Although we may be under the influence of the by-products of our previous attachments, aggression, and ignorance, this spark of intelligence includes a yearning for enlightenment; this yearning, though veiled by attachment, aggression, and ignorance will identify with whatever is necessary to bring into being whatever we think we are so that the process of unfolding the potential to enlightenment resumes. In the most basic terms, this means that consciousness becomes attracted to parents. As we move towards material form, the fourth nidana, we are conceived. And with conception our senses of hearing, smell, touch, taste as well as our feelings and thoughts emerge. These six are called the six-fold senses, the fifth nidana.

Up until this point, all of what has taken place is the direct result of previous experience, or past karma. Our previous attempts to resolve the Three Poisons leads us to experience our physical manifestation and its related sense fields in a particular way. Thus, as in Western medical science, at the time of conception our basic physical, mental/emotional, and spiritual predispositions (our rang-zhin) are established. Our body and senses will be impacted by attachment, aggression, and ignorance to the degree we have or have not resolved them in previous times. Still, our yearning for enlightenment, no matter how veiled with the illusions that arise from the Three Poisons, still exists. And although we are a product of our past karma, we possess an intelligence that recognizes the need to manifest in order to provide an opportunity to resolve whatever we have not resolved. This implies that at the point of conception, we are fully operational nascent beings who are beginning to deal with the world we find ourselves in. The development of the six-fold -

senses is the completion of what is produced by past karma. For it is at this point that we make contact with our present reality and start to develop our future karma.[4] We now have the physical capability to overtly react to further thought forms and impressions that arise in our minds and our embryonic environment. The interaction between the inner and outer reality has always been going on since they are one and the same thing: products of the mind classified as things within "me" or outside of "me." Beyond this basic distinction and how we find ourselves interacting with these phenomena as a result of the Three Poisons, we now have an opportunity to classify them further. The seventh nidana is called feeling, where we begin to have emotional reactions to that which we experience through our six-fold senses. How does something make us feel? Do we like it or dislike it? Does it make us happy, sad, or do we have no opinion about it whatsoever?

The next step, the eighth nidana, is to make discriminations as to what you want and what you wish to avoid. Now you are beginning to make choices, have overt reactions. Any pregnant mother will testify to the fact that she can feel, both psychologically and physically, when a baby likes or does not like what is coming into its environment, whether it be nourishment or some aspect of the environment.

With the intensity of discrimination arises a craving to obtain what one likes and to eliminate what one does not desire. This does not imply that what we crave is necessarily good for us. We can actually crave things that are injurious to us, but due to our ignorance and attachment we do not see the truth. Khenpo Rinpoche also teaches that craving can arise from fear of not having something. This is the origin of dependency and addiction.[5]

The more we get caught up in what we crave, the more mesmerized we become. We develop a psychological state of clinging, the ninth nidana, where we are so distracted by what we crave we actually believe that we could not exist without it. With our intentions focused in such a way, we create a context in which we ensure through our actions that we satisfy our cravings. Our willful intent is the tenth nidana, where there is no choice but the manifestation of things in accordance with our reactions to phenomena based on predispositions. The question here becomes whether we have exacerbated or resolved the Three Poisons in any way.

The eleventh nidana is called becoming or birth. This has to do with both psychological experience and physical birth since the nidanas operate in every moment of our existence as things are born and dissolve in our consciousness. We finally achieved that which we set out to achieve. It is a statement of all our desires bringing us to a point where the next logical step is to have to live out what has been created. Contrary to the notion that we are a tabula rasa, we emerge as a being with fairly well-established habits and preferences. We have created a predicament for ourselves that we now have to deal with as an independently functioning being.

The twelfth nidana concerns the law of cause and effect. What is created has limits. All things manifest, age, and die. The emotional ups and downs, the sicknesses we encounter, our interactions with the world around us, even our eventual demise—all of these circumstances we have set in motion. We may not be fully conscious of the implications of our life, but we cannot blame anyone else for the predicament we find ourselves in.

Because the twelve nidanas are a process we experience as we feel, discriminate, and make choices, it is possible to become more conscious of this process. If we do not recognize this process, the more solid and seemingly insoluble our world becomes; and the more separate from the world we appear to ourselves. The more materialistic we become, the more we view ourselves as machines. Thus, medically speaking, we run the risk of actually believing that it is a triviality to cut out organs, do transplants, add artificial organs or substances, or suppress our feelings by taking drugs, whether prescribed or not.

On the other hand, being able to recognize the twelve nidanas can be liberating as we begin to catch ourselves in the act of becoming fixated, spaced out, or aggressive. Although we cannot eliminate the twelve nidanas, since they are the natural process of the mind, for mindless, habitual responses that have negative outcomes we can substitute mindful responses that create the freedom for positive action and outcomes.

appendix two

THEORY OF THE THREE NYEPAS

Like many philosophies in the world, Ayurveda, as it is practiced in both the Indian and Tibetan traditions, classifies the cosmic and natural forces that are the basis for all that is manifest into a triad. Each branch of this triad is associated with specific gross physical properties and tendencies. The groupings of these properties and tendencies are as follows:

dry	unctuous	sticky
mobile	streaming	sluggish
subtle	piercing	stable
hard	liquidy	solid
rough	lustrous	wet
light	light	heavy
cool	hot	cool
vast		
penetrating		

All phenomena, animate or inanimate, possess these properties and tendencies in varying degrees. As they combine, all phenomena become imbued with structure or a varying degree of solidity, a varying degree of vibrancy, and a varying degree of molecular movement. Thus all things have structure, the potential to act in certain ways, and motion (whether visible or not). These attributes are classified as a function of the properties listed above.

ATTRIBUTE OF MOTION	motion	vibrancy (potency)	solidity (structural)

Asiatic cultures ascribe archetypal names to each branch of this primordial triad of properties, tendencies, and attributes. All three of these traditions speak of these three archetypal energy forms as the three humors. Listing them in the same order as in the columns above, these are:

(TIBETAN)	**LUNG** *(pronounced loong)*	**TrIPA** *(pronounced tee-pah)*	**BEKAN** *(pronounced bay-gahn*
(INDIAN OR SANSKRIT)	Vata	Pitta	Kapha
(CHINESE)	Chi	Yang	Yin

When translating the Tibetan humors, or nyepas—LUNG, TrIPA, and BEKAN—into the physical and psychological tendencies of animate creatures (such as humans), Tibetan and Western authorities on Tibetan medicine have used the term "wind" to mean LUNG, "bile" to mean TrIPA, and "phlegm" to mean BEKAN. Each of these substances does not, however, reflect the totality of what each humor represents in our constitutions.

All things in nature are conceived, are born, move through their life cycle, and die. In the Orient this process is seen in terms of five distinct transformations, or elements, in the process of life: ether, air, fire, water, and earth. Each humor is associated with two of these elements of life, the names of which are common in both Eastern and Western traditions.

LUNG = Ether and Air **TrIPA** = Fire and Water **BEKAN** = Water and Earth

Each of these pairs of elements is composed of opposites.

Ether is associated with creative potential. It is the space in which life is conceived. It is the impulse. It has the quality of being nontangible. As such, all potentials reside within it. Air is associated with maturity; life at its fullest. In this element, all of life finds its totality of manifestation. Ether (space) is filled by air. The two create a dynamic tension between being and nonbeing which expresses itself in the physical properties and tendencies of LUNG. This is considered the nontangible life force that exists within all things animate.

Fire is associated with gestation. It is the spark of life; what is coming into being is rich with a visible vibrancy. It is likened to the bud of a fruit or flower that possesses in its small, tight structure all the potential that will soon unfold. Water is associated with death or a state in which life is receding. Like sap going down into the roots of a tree in winter, it is a time of stillness. Life is a process of things growing and then disintegrating. By analogy, water can put out fire. The two combined create a dynamic tension, like a pressure cooker, bursting with potentiality, expressing the will to survive. They are the elements of TrIPA.

Earth is associated with solidity of form. It represents life at its densest, its most solid. This solidity provides protection and the certainty that as one moves towards maturity one has the strength to resist disintegrating forces and to nurture. Water represents fluidity. Water ensures that all of life will dissolve back into its constituent elements, whose potential will at some time in the future be revived. Earth absorbs water. It allows for the measured pace at which life comes and goes. The two create a dynamic tension that expresses itself in the physical properties and tendencies associated with BEKAN.

The archetypal forces of LUNG, TrIPA, and BEKAN and their associated elements represent more than just gross physical tendencies and traits or metaphors of life. These forces and their elements are the invisible energetic forces of creation that manifest themselves in the systems, structures, and functions of our physical body, our psychological character and emotional predisposition, and spiritual interests and inclinations.

The following chart provides a scheme of how each of our physical and mental/emotional characteristics and tendencies is classified according to the three humors, or nyepas.

CLASSIFICATION OF CHARACTERISTICS BASED ON THE THREE NYEPAS

HUMOR:	**LUNG**	**TrIPA**	**BEKAN**
ELEMENT:	Ether Air	Fire Water	Earth Water
PSYCHOLOGICAL FACULTY:	form and consciousness	conception and perception	feeling and perception
EMOTIONAL STATES:			
(balanced)	creative impulse, reflective interest, excitability	joy, cautious attentiveness	empathy, care, cautious attentiveness

(unbalanced)	irritability, nostalgia, frustration, rigid thinking, anger, passive aggression	anxiety, fear, paranoia, over-involvement, hysteria	sympathy, fear, paranoia, over-involvement, co-dependency
BODY TYPE (Western model)	ectomorph	mesomorph	endomorph
AREA OF BODY ASSOCIATED WITH	lower	middle	upper
SYSTEMS OF BODY	neurological psychological	endocrine vascular	digestive fluid systems (i.e., lymphatics)
PROMOTES:	mental health and awareness	immunity and vibrancy	physical stability and cleansing system
ASSOCIATED ORGANS	nervous system, heart, lungs, colon, skin, joints	small intestine, liver, gallbladder, veins, arteries, secretory organs, reproductive organs	stomach spleen/ pancreas, kidneys, bladder, lungs, lymph and lymph nodes
TYPES OF ILLNESSES (physical, examples)	cold illness (symptoms that move through the body), chronic lower G.I. tract problems (constipation), problems in associated organs	hot illness, infections, fevers, acute pains, endocrine and vascular problems, upper G. I. tract problems (diarrhea), problems in associated organs	cold illnesses, mucus and congestion, lethargy, low-grade and persistent pain, problems in associated organs
PRIMARY CAUSE OF DISORDER	attachment (becoming fixated or obsessed)	aggression (becoming overdiscerning, critical, or defensive)	ignorance (becoming lethargic about or not paying attention)

appendix three

A CONCISE MEDITATION ON MEDICINE BUDDHA

The following meditation is based on a traditional Tibetan Buddhist format and comes with the approval of H. E. Shamar Rinpoche. It can be done alone or with a group, read out loud or silently. The "pauses" mentioned in the text may be for any amount of time that you feel comfortable with.

Sitting in a manner that is calm, yet focused, we become aware of the formless passage of air as it comes in and passes from the tips of our noses. All distractions that arise in the mind are released with every natural exhalation.

(pause)

As we settle down into a state of centered awareness, we take some moments to **appreciate** the opportunity we have here and now.

(The Four Thoughts that turn the mind to spirituality)

We first recognize the **preciousness of our human birth**—where we have the time, circumstances, and capacity to learn from, practice the methods of, and experience the blessing of Enlightened Beings. Looking around us in the world and the difficult circumstances others have or experience, we appreciate how fortunate we are.

(pause)

Second, although this time, circumstance, and capacity is with us now, all can change in an instant and will certainly be gone at the moment of our death. There are no guarantees in this life other than the certainty that regardless of how stable our situation appears, we shall die. Appreciating **impermanence,** we resolve to use our human birth wisely.

(pause)

Third, we appreciate that the **causes and conditions** that give us this opportunity and will inevitably lead to their disappearing are the direct result of our own previous actions. Ultimately, we are the authors and masters of our own fate. We blame no one else for what we face and commit ourselves to taking responsibility for how we think and act in the moment. It is our thoughts and actions now that will determine what we shall have to face in our future.

(pause)

Finally, appreciating that we are masters of our own destiny and that our true potential is to be as a Buddha, we recognize the futility in placing any ultimate value on material and worldly pursuits and commit ourselves to a path of spiritual awakening for the benefit of all.

(pause)

(The Visualization)

And now, before us, out of the expanse of a clear turquoise-blue sky and just above the horizon, there arises the perfect form of the enlightened healer, the Medicine Buddha. Shimmering with the deep, rich color of crystalline lapis lazuli, He sits in the diamond (full lotus) posture, bearing all the marks and signs proclaiming His enlightened state and capacity to heal all afflictions. His rich, thick hair is tied up in a top knot and the simple maroon robes of a monk cover His powerful and dynamic body. His right hand rests on His right knee and between His thumb and index finger He holds the stem of the Arura, the king of medicinal plants. His left hand rests in His lap, holding a bowl filled with healing elixir. He sits, radiant, on a lotus throne supported by eight mighty, white lions. Having overcome all conditions that obstruct the realization of His full potential, His gaze is triumphant, yet kind. He is as real as anything, yet as insubstantial as everything—like a rainbow.

(Pause and allow the mind to settle on this visualization as clearly as possible.)

Looking upon the Medicine Buddha, we are inspired. Feeling confident in the unlimited capacity of His blessing and ability to heal, we think or say (three times),

To you, Teacher, Fully Aware Master and Adept, the Fully Awakened Lord of Healing, and King of Lapis Lazuli Light, I bow and open myself to the healing power of Your blessing.

We now recite the Medicine Buddha's mantra, the archetypal vibrations that help to eliminate all ignorance, attachment, and aggression, the Three Poisons that are at the root of all sufering.

We recite this mantra as many times as we can. As we do this, we see the Medicine Buddha's radiance (a rich, deep blue light) grow, reaching as far as we can imagine throughout all directions in space, bringing healing energy to each and every being it touches. At first we see this light go to friends and relatives for whom we are concerned, then everyone in general, and finally even to those we have difficulties with. **We include everyone in this blessing of radiance and healing.**

(Mantra)

TAY-YAH-TAH OM-BEH-KAHN-DZEH BEH-KAHN-DZEH MAH-HAH-BEH-KAHN-DZEH RAH-DZAH-SAH-MOOD-GAH-TAY SO-HAH

As we bring the recitation of mantras to a close, the Medicine Buddha before us comes closer and closer, dissolving into us through the crown of our heads. We now rest in a state where the illusion of separation between Medicine Buddha and ourselves vanishes. We remain in this state for as long as we can.

(pause)

When we recognize that our minds have become discursive once more, we instantly see our body, mind, and spirit as being none other than the Medicine Buddha. And, with this view we commit ourselves to behave in all matters as a Buddha. We **dedicate the merit** of this meditation in the spirit of the Diamond Way tradition by saying (aloud or to ourselves),

By practicing in this manner, may I quickly attain the realized state of the Medicine Buddha and, having done so, may I convert each and every being I meet into that same state.

With this new awareness of being inseparable and none other than the Medicine Buddha, slowly, in our own time, we become aware of the room and situation we find ourselves in here and now.

appendix four

MEWAS AND BUDDHIST SPIRITUAL PRACTICE

According to Tibetan Buddhist tradition, specific meditations are suggested to harmonize each of the mewas. The purpose or goal of each of these practices is expressed in general terms in the descriptions found in chapter 5. What follows are the suggested practices and mantras for those doing Tibetan Buddhist practice. At the same time, the mantras presented can be used by anyone with positive benefits.

ONE White Water

The meditation practice that is emphasized for the ONE White Water is that of Chenrezig or Loving Eyes. The mantra used is OM MANI PEME HUNG.

TWO Black Earth

The meditation practice that is suggested for the TWO Black Earth is performed for the purpose of clearing away obstacles. The deity is Chana Dorje and the mantra is OM BENZRA PANI HUNG.

THREE Blue Space

To overcome limitations and obstacles in the mind, the THREE Blue Space person is encouraged to meditate on Dorje Sempa or Diamond Mind and the mantra OM BENZRA SAHTO HUNG.

FOUR Green Space

To help the FOUR Green Space person overcome vulnerability and develop indestructible qualities, he or she is encouraged to meditate on Chana Dorje and recite the mantra OM BENZRA PANI HUNG.

FIVE Yellow Earth

The meditation practice suggested for the FIVE Yellow Earth person focuses on the Buddha Shakyamuni and his mantra OM MUNI MUNI MAHAMUNI SHAKYA MUNI YEH SOHA.

SIX White Air

The meditation practice for the SIX White Air person is intended for purification and to further longevity. The deity is Tsuk Tor Nam Gyal Ma and her mantra is OM AMRITA AYUR DADI SWAHA.

SEVEN Red Air

The meditation suggested is on the deity Green Tara, with her mantra OM TAREH TUTTAREH TUREH SOHA.

EIGHT White Earth

The suggested meditation practice for an EIGHT White Earth person is on Shakyamuni with his mantra, OM MUNI MUNI MAHAMUNI SHAKYAMUNI YEH SOHA.

NINE Maroon Fire

NINE Maroon Fire people are encouraged to meditate on the Bodhisattva of Wisdom, Manjusri, with his mantra OM AH RAH PAH TSAH NAH DHI.

NOTES

INTRODUCTION:

1. Terry Clifford, *Tibetan Buddhist Medicine and Psychiatry* (York Beach, Maine: Samuel Weiser, 1984), 48.

2. Yeshe Donden and Kelsang Jhampa, *Tibetan Medicine* (New Delhi, India: Library of Tibetan Works and Archives, 1977), preface.

3. Donden and Jhampa, *Tibetan Medicine*, 11. According to the tradition, the sage Yile Kye asks the sage Rigpe Yeshe of what the Ambrosia Heart Tantra is comprised. The sage Rigpe Yeshe enumerates and then goes into detail about the eight branches, eleven principles, fifteen divisions, and four compilations that are the basis of Tibetan medicine. The first, or Root Tantra, addresses the eight branches which discuss the types of illnesses that can be experienced by humans at different times of life and in different circumstances: "They are: (1) physical ailments, (2) children's ailments, (3) women's ailments, (4) men's ailments, (5) [ailments caused by] spirits, (6) [wounds afflicted by] weapons, (7) [disorders of the] aged and (8) sterility." The second, or Explanatory Tantra, talks about the eleven principles which help people remain free of illness. These include such topics as anatomy and physiology, sound nutritional and behavioral practices, and the role and behavior of a physician. The third, the Oral Tradition Tantra, enumerates the fifteen divisions on how to use specific cures for specific illnesses. The final, or Subsequent Tantra, deals with in-depth diagnosis and medical intervention, such as methods of inducing the various forms of bodily elimination, moxabustion, even surgery. According to Terry Clifford's *Tibetan Buddhist Medicine and Psychiatry*, there are 156 chapters of detailed medical information presented in the *Gyud-Zhi*.

4. Clifford, *Tibetan Buddhist Medicine and Psychiatry*, 48.

5. Leon Hammer, *Dragon Rises, Red Bird Flies* (Barrytown, N.Y.: Station Hill Press, 1991).

CHAPTER 1: SELF-EVALUATION

1. Please note that the Three Poisons also go by other names in other reliable sources for Tibetan medicine and philosophy. Attachment is also referred to as desire, passion, clinging, even lust. Aggression is referred to as aversion, hatred, or anger. Ignorance is referred to as delusion, obscuration, or confusion. These variations in names do not alter what nyepa they are associated with. See Dr. Yeshe Donden's *Health through Balance*, Dr. Tom Dummer's *Tibetan Medicine*, and Terry Clifford's *Tibetan Buddhist Medicine and Psychiatry*, all cited in the Bibliography.

2. See also chart, pages 215–16.

3. Ideally, to determine the patient's rang-zhin, a Tibetan doctor would want to have the following conditions met:

(1) The patient must be able to have two weeks of normal, natural activity during which there are no extraordinary events, i.e., travel, festivals, and so forth.

(2) The patient eats a simple diet of rice, dahl, and vegetables. The purpose of this is to sustain the body but avoid overstimulation through such things as meat and alcohol.

(3) The patient would take a written or an oral test assessing his or her psychological predisposition and personal habits, after following the dietary and activity regimen indicated in 1 and 2, above.

(4) Upon rising on the day of the medical examination, the patient produces a midstream sample of urine in a clean vessel for inspection by the physician. The patient does not eat anything before the examination.

(5) At the examination, the physician carefully observes the patient's frame, physiognomy, tongue, eyes, and fingernails. The urine is examined in terms of its color, smell, taste, and frothiness. There is even a divination process that is done with the urine as medium.

(6) Astrological data are studied.

(7) A history is taken of the patient's illnesses and those of his or her immediate family (parents and grandparents). The patient also describes his or her daily regimen.

(8) The physician takes the various pulses to determine nyepa dominance, the condition of the various organs, and which nyepa is influencing their function.

(9) Compiling all of the above data, the physician determines the patient's rang-zhin.

In the modern world, few of us would find a Tibetan or Ayurvedic physician, let alone be able to fulfill such ideal requirements. Of course, it is well worth the effort to obtain such an accurate determination of one's rang-zhin.

4. Yeshe Donden, *Health Through Balance* (Ithaca, N.Y.: Snow Lion Publications, 1986), 77.

5. Ibid., 80.

6. Dr. Vasant Lad, 1987 lecture series.

7. Tai Situ Rinpoche, *Relative World, Ultimate Mind* (Boston and London: Shambhala Publications, 1992).

CHAPTER 2: NUTRITIONAL PRACTICES

1. Ivan Illich, *Medical Nemesis—The Expropriation of Health* (New York: Pantheon Books, 1976).

2. Yeshe Donden and Kelsang Jhampa, *Tibetan Medicine (The Ambrosia Heart Tantra)* (New Delhi, India: Library of Tibetan Works and Archives, 1977), 90.

3. Lino Stanchich, *The Power Eating Program* (Miami, Fla.: Healthy Products, 1989).

4. Rechung Rinpoche, *Tibetan Medicine* (Berkeley and Los Angeles: University of California Press, 1976), 63.

5. Yeshe Donden, *Health Through Balance* (Ithaca, N.Y.: Snow Lion Publications, 1986), 170.

6. Ibid.

7. John Robbins, *Diet for a New America* (Walpole, N.H.: Stillpoint Publishing, 1987).

8. Hazel R. Parcells, *For Better Health*.(Albuquerque, New Mexico: Parcells System of Scientific Living, Inc., 1989).

9. Ibid., p.6.

10. Khenpo Karthar, Rinpoche, *Medicine Buddha Commentary*, (Woodstock, New York: Karma Triyana Dharmachakra, 1984), 50.

11. Rechung Rinpoche, *Tibetan Medicine*, 61.

12. Ibid.

13. Ibid.

14. Ilza Veith, *Yellow Emperor Classics of Internal Medicine*.(Berkley, Los Angeles, London: University of California Press, 1972).

15. Tom Dummer, *Tibetan Medicine and Other Holistic Health-Care Systems* (London and New York: Routledge, 1988), 97.

16. Ibid., 57–58

17. Amadea Morningstar, *The Ayurvedic Cookbook* (Santa Fe, N.M.: Lotus Press, 1990), 29.

18. Ibid.

19. Amadea Morningstar, lecture at Ayurvedic Institute, 1987.

20. Dr. Lobsang Rapgay, 1988 lecture series.

21. Rechung Rinpoche, *Tibetan Medicine*, 63.

22. Donden, *Health through Balance*, 154.

CHAPTER 3: EXERCISE

1. Yeshe Donden and Kelsang Jhampa, *Tibetan Medicine (The Ambrosia Heart Tantra)* (New Delhi, India: Library of Tibetan Works and Archives, 1977), 85.

2. Terry Clifford, *Tibetan Buddhist Medicine and Psychiatry* (York Beach, Maine: Samuel Weiser, 1984), 212.

3. Yeshe Donden, *Health Through Balance* (Ithaca, N.Y.: Snow Lion Publications, 1986), 182.

4. Tarthang Tulku, *Kum Nye Relaxation, Part 1: Theory, Preparation, Massage* (Berkeley, Calif.: Dharma Publishing, 1978), x.

5. Ibid., 7–8

6. Unpublished essay "Exercise and Ayurveda" by Melanie Sachs.

7. Peter Kelder, *Ancient Secrets of the Fountain of Youth* (Gig Harbor, Wa.: Harbor Press, 1985).

8. Christopher S. Kilham, *Inner Power: Secrets from Tibet and the Orient* (Tokyo and New York: Japan Publications, 1988).

9. Ibid., 78.

10. Kelder, *Fountain of Youth*, 24.

11. Unpublished manuscript by Dr. Lobsang Rapgay, 117.

12. Dr. Lobsang Rapgay, 1988 seminar.

CHAPTER 4: Skillful Behavior

1. Yeshe Donden and Kelsang Jhampa, *Tibetan Medicine (The Ambrosia Heart Tantra)* (New Delhi, India: Library of Tibetan Works and Archives, 1977), 84.

2. Terry Clifford, *Tibetan Buddhist Medicine and Psychiatry* (York Beach, Maine: Samuel Weiser, 1984), 99.

3. Donden, *Tibetan Medicine*, 85.

4. Vasant Lad, *Ayurveda: The Science of Self Healing* (Santa Fe, N.M.: Lotus Press, 1984), 100.

5. Rechung Rinpoche, *Tibetan Medicine* (Berkeley and Los Angeles: University of California Press, 1976), 54.

6. Clifford, *Tibetan Buddhist Medicine and Psychiatry*, 141.

7. Gedun Chopel, *Tibetan Arts of Love* (Ithaca, N.Y.: Snow Lion Publications, 1992), 230.

8. Nik Douglas and Penny Slinger, *Sexual Secrets*, (Vermont: Destiny Books, 1979), 251.

9. Kalu Rinpoche, *The Gem Ornament of Manifold Oral Instructions* (San Francisco: KDK Publications, 1986), 99.

10. Yeshe Donden, *Health Through Balance* (Ithaca, N.Y.: Snow Lion Publications, 1986), 143.

11. Dharmaraksita, *The Wheel of Sharp Weapons* (New Delhi, India: Library of Tibetan Works and Archives, 1981), 17.

12. Donden, *Tibetan Medicine*, 89.

13. Ibid., 93.

CHAPTER 5: Meditation and Spiritual Practice

1. Dr. Lobsang Rapgay, lecture, 1988.

2. Bob Sachs, *The Complete Guide to Nine-Star Ki* (Shaftesbury, England: Element Press, 1992).

3. Ibid., 93.

4. Ibid., 85.

5. Ibid., 77–78.

6. Ibid., 70.

7. Ibid., 62.

8. Ibid., 55–56.

9. Ibid., 48–49.

10. Ibid., 43.

11. Ibid., 37.

12. Chogyam Trungpa, Rinpoche, *Shambhala: Sacred Path of the Warrior* (Boulder, Colo.: Shambhala Publications, 1973), 60.

CHAPTER 6: DETOXIFICATION AND REJUVENATION

1. Very Venerable Chogyam Trungpa, Rinpoche, lecture at Woodstock Town Hall, 1979.

2. Ayurvedic Learning Center, Santa Fe, New Mexico, brochure, 1991.

3. Dr. Lobsang Rapgay, in conversation, 1988.

4. Dr. Sunil Joshi, lecture, fall 1990.

5. Hara Shiatsu International Newsletter (Winter 1988–1989), 7.

6. Ibid.

7. Dr. Patrick Hanaway, in conversation, fall 1992.

8. Terry Clifford, *Tibetan Buddhist Medicine and Psychiatry* (York Beach, Maine: Samuel Weiser, 1984), 185.

9. Dr. Sunil Joshi, lecture, fall 1990.

10. Dr. Lobsang Rapgay, lecture series, 1988.

11. Venerable Khenpo Karthar, Rinpoche, presentation, 1990.

12. Yeshe Donden, *Health Through Balance* (Ithaca, N.Y.: Snow Lion Publishing, 1986), 207-213.

CHAPTER 7: TIME AND PLACE

1. Tai Situ Rinpoche, *Relative World, Ultimate Mind* (Boston and London: Shambhala Publications, 1992), 108.

2. Ibid., 8–9.

3. Sarah Rossbach, *Feng Shui: The Chinese Art of Placement* (New York: E. P. dutton, 1983).

4. Tai Situ Rinpoche, *Relative World, Ultimate Mind*, 97.

5. Matrix Software Tibetan Astrology Seminar, preliminary notes.

6. Dr. Lobsang Rapgay, lecture series, 1988.

APPENDIX ONE

1. Tai Situ Rinpoche in Maitreya Institute lecture.

2. Heart Sutra.

3. Venerable Khenpo Karthar, Rinpoche, lecture, 1978.

4. Ibid.

GLOSSARY

BEKAN (Tibetan). (Sanskrit: *kapha*). The humor, or *nyepa*, of phlegm, one of the three main constituents of the body. In Chinese it is associated with the yin force. It has to do with all that is sticky and solid within the body, basically structure and lubrication. Its seat is in the stomach. It is associated with the mental poison of ignorance, which when transformed, becomes the vast mind of enlightenment.

Dzub-nyin (Tibetan). (Japanese: *shiatsu*). Acupressure-type massage.

Jamtsi (Tibetan). (Sanskrit: *basti*). Therapeutic enema intended to both clean and rejuvenate the colon.

Kar-tse (Tibetan). Astrology. An astrologer is a *kar-tsepa*.

Kyuk (Tibetan). (Sanskrit: *vomina*). Emetic.

Len Nga (Tibetan) therapy. (Sanskrit: *Pancha Karma*). Literally meaning "five actions" intended to rid the body of excesses, restore balance, and slow, if not reverse, the aging process. Includes massages, steams, digestive tract cleansing processes, nasal administrations, and other special techniques.

LUNG (Tibetan, pronounced 'loong'). (Sanskrit: *vata*). Known as the humor, or nyepa, of wind, one of the three primary constituents of all forms in creation. Also called the life force (or *chi* in Chinese) which moves all substances and is the source of all actions in the body. Its seat is in the colon, and it is associated particularly with the nervous system and our psychological makeup. Associated with the mental poison of attachment, which once transformed, creates compassion and allows us to experience our mind as unimpeded.

Marma (Sanskrit). Neuro-lymphatic points used in various forms of massage in both India and Tibet. Literally translated, *marma* means a point that can kill. Some of these points are common in the martial arts. The ones used for healing are touched very lightly and have profound effects on the organs and functions they are associated with. If they are damaged through injury or surgical intervention, they can be the cause of chronic, irresolvable health conditions that will need ongoing attention.

Mewa (Tibetan). Literally means birthmark and is an aspect of Tibetan astrology. The *mewa* is represented by a number and associated element. There is a mewa for each year, and its characteristics are an important part of understanding a person's character and spiritual inclinations.

Na Jong (Tibetan). (Sanskrit: *nasya*). Nasal administration of oils or herbs.

Netra Basti (Sanskrit). Bathing the eyes in clarified butter.

Nyepa (Tibetan). (Sanskrit: *dosha*). Humor of the body dominated by one of the Three Poisons (ignorance, attachment, aggression). Each nyepa has associated functions, tissues, and psychological predispositions.

Pho thut (Tibetan). (Sanskrit: *agni*). Digestive fire.

Rang-zhin (Tibetan). (Sanskrit: *prakruti*). Constitution, basic strengths and weaknesses as determined at conception. It is relatively unchangeable and determines what health-care and spiritual practices are best for our growth and development.

Sache (Tibetan). (Chinese: *feng shui*). Geomancy, or the art of placement; understanding how the positioning of objects and features in natural and man-made environments affect our well-being.

Shirodhara (Sanskrit). A *Len Nga* therapeutic process whereby warm sesame oil is poured slowly on the crown of the head while sitting up (Tibetan-style) or lying on one's back with the oil pouring onto the region of the third eye (Indian style).

Sok-lung (Tibetan). (Sanskrit: *prana*). The subtle but necessary aspect of our life force.

Three Poisons. The three dominant mental disturbances (ignorance, attachment, and aggression) that are the root causes of all suffering, be it mental or physical. They are the roots of all manifest form, including the human body, and it is the goal of Tibetan medicine to bring their manifestations into balance so that spiritual practice can transform the poisons into enlightened awareness and action.

TrIPA (Tibetan). (Sanskrit: *pitta*). One of the nyepas, or humors, often called fire, or bile, and one of the three main constituents of all things in creation. In Chinese it is associated with the yang force. This is associated with all that is transformed in body and mind. Common associations are metabolism, endocrine functioning, and all organs associated with these processes. Its seat is the small intestine. The mental poison associated with it is aggression, which, when transformed, gives us a sense clarity and joy.

Twelve Nidanas. The Buddhist doctrine of interdependent origination, the process by which thoughts arise and become manifestations and seeds for future thoughts and subsequent manifestations; better known as karma.

BIBLIOGRAPHY

TIBETAN AND AYURVEDIC MEDICINE

Chopra, Dr. Deepak. *Perfect Health*. New York: Harmony Books, 1991.

Clifford, Terry. *Tibetan Buddhist Medicine and Psychiatry*. York Beach, Maine: Samuel Weiser, 1984.

Donden, Dr. Yeshe. *Health Through Balance*. Ithaca, New York: Snow Lion Publications, 1986.

Donden, Dr. Yeshe, and Kelsang Jhampa. *Tibetan Medicine (The Ambrosia Heart Tantra)*. New Delhi, India: Library of Tibetan Works and Archives, 1977.

Dummer, Tom. *Tibetan Medicine and Other Holistic Health-Care Systems*. London and New York: Routledge, 1988.

Joshi, Dr. Sunil V. *Ayurveda and Panchakarma: The Science of Healing and Rejuvenation*. Twin Lakes, Wis.: Lotus Press, 1997.

Kurian, Joseph. *Living in Beauty*. San Francisco: EMC Publishing, 2000.

Lad, Dr. Vasant. *Ayurveda: The Science of Self-Healing*. Santa Fe, N.M.: Lotus Press, 1984.

Ranade, Ranade, Qutab, and Deshpande. *Health and Disease in Ayurveda and Yoga*. Maharashtra, India: Anmol Prakashan, 1997.

Rapgay, Dr. Lobsang. *The Tibetan Book of Healing*. Salt Lake City, Utah: Passage Press, 1997.

———. *Tibetan Medicine: A Holistic Approach to Better Health*. New Delhi, India: Indraprastha Press, 1985.

Venerable Rechung Rinpoche. *Tibetan Medicine*. Berkeley and Los Angeles: University of California Press, 1976.

Thakkur, Chandrashekhar G. *Introduction to Ayurveda*. Bombay, India: The Times of India Press, 1965.

CHINESE MEDICINE

Veith, Ilza (editor). *The Yellow Emperor's Classic of Internal Medicine*. Berkeley, Los Angeles, and London: University of California Press, 1972.

NUTRITION AND HERBS

Ballentine, Dr. Rudolph. *Diet and Nutrition*. Honesdale, Pa.: The Himalayan International, 1978.

Bragg, Ginna Bell, and Dr. David Simon. *A Simple Celebration*. New York: Harmony Books, 1997.

Colbin, Annemarie. *Food and Healing*. New York: Ballentine Books, 1986.

Gagne, Stephen. *Energetics of Food*. Santa Fe, N.M.: Spiral Sciences, 1990.

Lad, Usha, and Dr. Vasant Lad. *Ayurvedic Cooking for Self-Healing*. Albuquerque, N.M.: The Ayurvedic Press, 1994.

Lad, Dr. Vasant, and David Frawley. *The Yoga of Herbs*. Santa Fe, N.M.: Lotus Press, 1986.

Morningstar, Amadea. *The Ayurvedic Cookbook*. Santa Fe, N.M.: Lotus Press, 1990.

———. *Ayurvedic Cooking for Westerners*. Twin Lakes, Wis.: Lotus Press, 1995.

Robbins, John. *Diet for a New America*. Walpole, N.H.: Stillpoint Publishing, 1987.

Singha, Dr. Shyam. *The Secrets of Natural Health*. Shaftesbury, England: Element Press, 1997.

Stanchich, Lino. *The Power Eating Program*. Miami, Fla.: Healthy Products, 1989.

Svoboda, Dr. Robert. *Prakruti*. Albuquerque, N.M.: Geocom Ltd., 1988.

Tierra, Dr. Michael. *Planetary Herbology*. Santa Fe, N.M.: Lotus Press, 1988.

EXERCISE AND RELAXATION

Chia, Mantak, and Maneewan Chia. *Awaken Healing Light of the Tao*. Huntington, N.Y.: Healing Tao Books, 1993.

Frawley, Dr. David. *Yoga and Ayurveda*. Twin Lakes, Wis.: Lotus Press, 1999.

Kelder, Peter. *Ancient Secrets of the Fountain of Youth.* Gig Harbor, Wash.: Harbor Press, 1985.
Kilham, Christopher S. *Inner Power: Secrets from Tibet and the Orient.* Tokyo and New York: Japan Publications, 1988.
Norbu, Namkhai. *Yantra Yoga.* Gleisdorf, Germany: Tsaparang, 1988.
Reed Gach, Michael. *Acu-Yoga.* Tokyo and New York: Japan Publications, 1981.
Sutton, Dr. Marcea. *In Harmony: Resolving Stress.* Albuquerque, N.M.: Zivah Publishers, 1991.
Tarthang Tulku. *Kum Nye Relaxation, Part 1: Theory, Preparation, Massage.* Berkeley, Calif.: Dharma Publishing, 1978.

SEXUAL BEHAVIOR AND PRACTICES

Chang, Jolan. *The Tao of Sex and Love.* New York: E. P. Dutton, 1977.
Chia, Mantak. *Taoist Secrets of Love.* Santa Fe, N.M.: Aurora Press, 1984.
Chia, Mantak, and Maneewan Chia. *Healing Love through the Tao.* Huntington, N.Y.: Healing Tao Books, 1986.
Chopel, Gedun. *Tibetan Arts of Love.* Ithaca, N.Y.: Snow Lion Publications, 1992.

MEDITATION AND SPIRITUAL PRACTICE

Birnbaum, Raoul. *The Healing Buddha.* Boulder, Colo.: Shambhala Publications, 1979.
Dharmaraksita. *The Wheel of Sharp Weapons.* New Delhi, India: Library of Tibetan Works and Archives, 1981.
Fremantle, Francesca, and Chogyam Trungpa. *The Tibetan Book of the Dead.* Boulder, Colo., and London: Shambhala Publications, 1975.
Kalu Rinpoche. *The Gem Ornament of Manifold Oral Instructions.* San Francisco: KDK Publications, 1986.
———. *The Dharma.* Albany, N.Y.: State University of New York Press, 1986.
Khenpo Karthar Rinpoche. *Dharma Paths.* Ithaca, N.Y.: Snow Lion Publications, 1992.
Lati, Rinpoche, and Jeffrey Hopkins. *Death, Intermediate State and Rebirth in Tibetan Buddhism.* Ithaca, N.Y.: Snow Lion Publications, 1985.
Nyadahl, Lama Ole. *Teachings on the Nature of the Mind.* Nevada City, Calif.: Blue Dolphin Publishing, 1993.
Sogyal Rinpoche. *The Tibetan Book of Living and Dying.* San Francisco and New York: Harper, 1992.
Tai Situ Rinpoche. *Relative World, Ultimate Mind.* Boston and London: Shambhala Publications, 1992.
Trungpa, Chogyam. *Shambhala: The Sacred Path of the Warrior.* Boulder, Colo.: Shambhala Publications, 1984.
———. *Cutting through Spiritual Materialism.* Boulder, Colo., and London: Shambhala Publications, 1973.
Wangyal, Tenzin. *The Tibetan Yogas of Dream and Sleep.* Ithaca, N.Y.: Snow Lion Publications, 1998.

MASSAGE AND AYURVEDIC TREATMENTS

Johari, Harish. *Ayurvedic Massage: Traditional Indian Techniques for Balancing Body and Mind.* Rochester, Vt.: Healing Arts Press, 1996.
Joshi, Dr. Sunil V. *Ayurveda and Panchakarma: The Science of Healing and Rejuvenation.* Twin Lakes, Wis.: Lotus Press, 1997.
Rapgay, Dr. Lobsang. *Tibetan Therapeutic Massage.* New Delhi, India: Indraprastha Press, 1985.
Sachs, Melanie. *Ayurvedic Beauty Care.* Santa Fe, N.M.: Lotus Press, 1994.

ASTROLOGY, GEOMANCY, AND DIVINATION

Cornu, Philippe. *Tibetan Astrology.* Boston and London: Shambhala, 1997.
Goldberg, Jay, Doya Nardin, and Mipham Nardin. *Mo: Tibetan Divination System.* Ithaca, N.Y.: Snow Lion Publications, 1990.

Lassalle, Rex. *Grasshopping through Time*. London: Rex Lassalle, 1998.
Lim, Dr. Jes T. Y. *Feng Shui and Your Health*. Singapore: Time Books International, 1999.
Rossbach, Sarah. *Feng Shui: The Chinese Art of Placement*. New York: E. P. Dutton, 1983.
Sachs, Robert. *Nine Star Ki: Your Astrological Companion to Feng Shui*. Shaftesbury, England: Element Books, 1999.
Sandifer, Jon. *Feng Shui Astrology: Using Nine Star Ki to Achieve Harmony and Happiness*. London, England: Piatkus Press, 1997.
Simons, T. Raphael. *Feng Shui Step by Step*. New York: Three Rivers Press, 1996.
Spear, William. *Feng Shui Made Easy*. San Francisco: HarperCollins, 1995.
Walters, Derek. *Chinese Astrology*. Wellingborough, England: The Aquarian Press, 1987.
Wangchuck, Sangye. "Matrix Software Tibetan Astrology Seminar." Big Rapids, Mich.: Matrix Software, 1988 (unpublished).

RESOURCES

TO STUDY TIBETAN MEDICINE AND CONTACT TIBETAN DOCTORS:

Dr. Yeshi Donden
"Ashok Niwas"
McLeod Ganj.
Dharamsala,
Distt. Kangra,
H.P. India

Dr. Tenzin Choedhak and Staff Physicians
Tibetan Medical and Astro Institute
Khara Danda Road
Dharamsala,
Distt. Kangra
(Himal Pradesh)
India

Dr. Lobsang Rapgay
2206 Benecia Avenue
Westwood, CA 90064
(310) 282-9918

Chagpori Tibetan Medical Institute
(Dr. Trogawa)
Trogawa House
P.O. North Point
Darjeeling 734 104
W.B. India

Dr. Barry Clark
c/o Library of Tibetan Works and Archives
Gangchen Kyishong
Dharamsala
Distt. Kangra,
H.P. India

Shakya Dorje
(416) 234-9199

New World Medical Center
Dr. Marsha Woolf
416 West 23rd, Suite 1D
New York, NY 10011
(212) 741-2727/(508) 336-8787

Chakpori Institute
(Principle physician: Dr. Trogawa)
151-31 88th Street, Box 2D
Howard Beach, NY 11414
(718) 641-7323

Diamond Way Ayurveda
(Preventive Health-Care Education: Robert Sachs)
P.O. Box 13753
San Luis Obispo, CA 93406
(877) 964-1395
Fax: (805)543-9291
E-mail: diamond.way.ayurveda@thegrid.net

TO STUDY AYURVEDIC MEDICINE:

Ayurvedic Health Center
2509 Virginia N.E., Suite D
Albuquerque, NM 87110
(505) 296-6522

The Ayurvedic Institute and Wellness Center
P.O. Box 23445
Albuquerque, NM 87192-1445
(505) 291-9698

Ayurvedic Living Workshops
P.O. Box 188
Exeter, Devon EX4 5AB
England

California College of Ayurveda
135 Argall Way
Nevada City, CA 95959
(916) 265-4300

Diamond Way Ayurveda
P.O. Box 13753
San Luis Obispo, CA 93406
(877) 964-1395

Lotus Ayurvedic Center
4145 Clares Street, Suite D
Capitola, CA 95010
(408) 479-1667

Natural Therapeutics Center
"Surya Daya"
Gisingham, Nr. Iye
Suffolk, England

Twenty-first Century Medical Center
111 Elm Street, Suite 104
Worcester, MA 01609-1967
(508) 753-0006
Fax: (508) 770-0618

Wise Earth Institute
Attn. Bri Maya Tiwari
27–29 Tacoma Place
Asheville, NC 28800

CORRESPONDENCE COURSE:

American Institute of Vedic Studies
Attn. David Frawley
P.O. Box 8357
Santa Fe, NM 87504
(505) 983-9385

TO GET TIBETAN HERBS, PRECIOUS PILLS, AND SUPPLIES:

Diamond Way Ayurveda
P.O. Box 13753
San Luis Obispo, CA 93406
Telephone or Fax: (805) 543-9291
(877) 964-1395
www.DiamondWayAyurveda.com

Karma Herbs
c/o Dr. Lobsang Rapgay
2206 Benecia Avenue
Westwood, CA 90064
(310) 282-9918

Tibetan Medical and Astro Institute
Khara Danda Road
Dharamsala - 176215
Distt. Kangra
H.P. India

Kunphen Tibetan Medical Hall and Clinic
15/22 Chhetrapati
Kathmandu, Nepal

TO GET AYURVEDIC HERBS AND SUPPLIES:

The Ayurvedic Institute and Wellness Center
11311 Menaul N.E., Suite A
Albuquerque, NM 87112
(505) 291-9698

Ayush Herbs, Inc.
10025 N.E. 4th Street
Bellevue, WA 98004
(800) 925-1371

Banyan Trading Company
P.O. Box 13002
Albuquerque, NM 87192
(800) 953-6424
Fax: (505) 244-1878

Bazaar of India Imports, Inc.
1810 University Avenue
Berkeley, CA 94703
(510) 548-4110

Herbalvedic Products
P.O. Box 6054
Santa Fe, NM 87502

Lotus Brands, Inc.
P.O. Box 325
Twin Lakes, WI 53181

Lotus Herbs
1505 42nd Avenue, Suite 19
Capitola, CA 95010
(408) 479-1667

TO STUDY TAI CHI:

Garuda School Tibetan Tai Chi
10900 Menaul N.E.
Albuquerque, NM 87112
(505) 292-6868
(Instructor: Marilyn Feeney)

TO STUDY KUM NYE EXERCISE:

Nyingma Institute
2425 Hillside Avenue
Berkeley, CA 94704

TO STUDY YANTRA YOGA:

Dzogchen Community West Coast
P.O. Box 20781
Oakland, CA 94620

Tsegyalgar Dzogchen Community
Parsons Street
Conway, MA 01341

Dzogchen Community of England
c/o John Renshaw
14D Chesterton Road
London W10 5XL
England

Comunita Dzogchen Merigar
58031 Arcidosso (GR)
Italy

TO RECEIVE TIBETAN ASTROLOGICAL CHARTS:
(Send your name, with date, hour, and place of birth, and $35 money order)

Tibetan Astrological Service
P.O. Box 7
Hay-on-Wye
Hereford, HR3 5TU
England

(For Sangye Wangchuck's astrological materials and Tibetan Buddhist calendars)

Matrix Software
315 Marion Avenue
Big Rapids, MI 49307

FOR NINE-STAR KI ASTROLOGY CHARTS:

Robert Sachs
Diamond Way Ayurveda
P.O. Box 13753
San Luis Obispo, CA 93406
Telephone or Fax: (805) 543-9291
Web site: www.NineStarKi.net

TO ORDER CALENDARS:

(TIBETAN—BASED ON LUNAR CYCLE OF DAYS)
Rigpa
449 Powell Street, Suite 200
San Francisco, CA 94102
(415) 392-2055
Fax: (415) 392-2056
Web site: www.rigpa.org

(NINE-STAR KI OR MEWA AND ANIMAL DAY CHARTS)
J. Koji-Higa
9 Ki Resources
P.O. Box 638
Great Barrington, MA 01230
(413) 528-3260
E-mail: nineki@juno.com

FOR INFORMATION ABOUT MEDITATION INSTRUCTION AND CLASSES:
The following organizations can provide you with local or regional contact persons and/or center.

(NONDENOMINATIONAL)
Shambhala Training International
Executive Offices
1084 Tower Road
Halifax, Nova Scotia
Canada B3H 265

(KAGYU SECT OF TIBETAN BUDDHISM)
Diamond Way Buddhist Centers
110 Merced Avenue
San Francisco, CA 94127
(415) 661-6467
Fax: (415) 665-2241
Web site: www.diamondway-buddhism.org

Karma Triyana Dharmachakra
352 Meads Mountain Road
Woodstock, NY 12498

Kagyu Shepen Kunchah Buddhist Center
751 Airport Road
Santa Fe, NM 87501

(SAKYA SECT OF TIBETAN BUDDHISM)
Sakya Center
P.O. Box 606
Porter Square Station
Cambridge, MA 02140

(NYINGMA SECT OF TIBETAN BUDDHISM)
The Vajrayana Foundation
531 Corralitos Road, Suite 108
Corralitos, CA 95076

(GELUG SECT OF TIBETAN BUDDHISM)
Namgyal Monastery
Institute of Buddhist Studies
P.O. Box 127
Ithaca, NY 14851

(BON TRADITION)
The Ligmincha Institute
P.O. Box 1892
Charlottesville, VA 22903
(804) 977-6161
Fax: (804) 977-7020
E-mail: ligmincha@aol.com

Tibetan Bon Temple Foundation
2020 Stanley Avenue
Signal Hill, CA 90806

(ALL TRADITIONS)
Snow Lion Publications
P.O. Box 6483
Ithaca, NY 14851

TIBETAN MEDICAL PROJECTS THAT NEED SUPPORT:

Karma Thegsum Tashi Gomang Medical Project
Box 39
Crestone, CO 81131
(719) 256-4695
(Contact: Marianne Marstrand)

Chakpori Institute
(Principle physician: Dr. Trogawa)
151–31 88th Street, Box 2D
Howard Beach, NY 11414
(718) 641-7323

INDEX

abdomen, 169
abdominal muscles, 105, 107, 109
acid rain, 80
acupressure, 123, 181, 239
acupuncture, 17, 22
acupuncture points, 169
addiction, 127, 211
adultery, 127
aerobics, 95, 96
age factors, 49
aggression, 26–28, 30, 95, 119, 215–22, 233n.1, 239, 240
aggression/anger, 164
aging. *See* rejuvenation
agitation, 144
agni, 58, 75, 89–92, 240
agrarian, 54
air, 80–81, 224–25
alcohol, 32, 136, 175
alcoholic hangovers, 123
alienation, 26
allergies, 90, 137
allopathy, 12, 54, 165
alpha brain waves, 113–15, 118, 121, 143, 184
alternative health-care models, 12, 16, 19, 53, 165, 171
altruism, 131–33
Ambrosia Heart Tantra, The. *See Gyud–Zhi*
Ancient Indian Massage (Johari), 168–69
Ancient Secrets of the Fountain of Youth (Kelder), 102, 109–10, 111
anemia, 173
anger/aggression, 164
animal proteins, 74
animal signs, 199–203
animals, domesticated, 76
antagonistic days, 201–204
antibiotics, 54, 76
antidepressants, 190
antidotes to meditation problems, 161–64
antihistamines, 54
archetypal names, 223–24
arthritis, 53
artificial organs, 222
asfoetida, 162
asthma, 174
astringent, 55
astrology, 11–12, 153–61, 197, 198–204, 213, 239
attachment, 26–28, 29, 47, 119, 215–22, 233n.l, 239, 240
attention deficit disorder, 181
autumn, 137
awakened state of being, 167, 217
awareness, 27, 240
Ayurveda, Tibetan, 25–26, 47, 166
Ayurvedic Beauty Care (Sachs), 101, 124, 136
Ayurvedic Center of Santa Fe, New Mexico, 167
Ayurvedic Cookbook, The (Morningstar), 58, 75, 91
Ayurvedic health practitioners, 32

baboons, 76
back pain, 90
barley flour, 58
basketball, 96
basmas, 85–86
basti, 223
baths, 123, 124, 136, 169
bay, 169
bean flours, 170
bears, black, 77
beauty, 13
becoming, 222
beets, 75
behavior, skillful, 119–40
"being present," 143
BEKAN, 28, 30–31, 50, 223–26, 239; and climate, 19; and digestive fire, 91; and exercise, 93, 96; food recommendations for, 66–69; and leftovers, 75–76; *Len Nga* process for, 187; massage for, 169; and relaxation, 118; and seasons, 135, 137; and sex, 129; and sleep, 122; and stomach, 171; and tastes, 55; and vomiting, 173–74
belching, 90
beverages, 90, 96, 136
bile, 77, 224, 240

biofeedback, 114, 118
bird, 200–204
birth and karma, 216–22
birth year, 153
birthmark, 153, 239
bitter, 55
black bears, 77
blaming, 147
Blank, Ivy, 167
blemish, 153
blood and nerve cleansing, 177–78
blood donations, 131
bloodletting, 22
bloodlines, 166, 188
bodhisattvas, 29, 31, 51
body agility, 167
body chemistry, 21
body mandala, 113
body postures, 113
body sensation and relaxation, 115
body systems of *nyepas*, 226
body types of *nyepas*, 226
bodybuilding, 95
body-mind-spirit integration, 17, 25–26, 52 99–100, 167
Bonner, Thomas, 13
Bonpo shamanism, 22
bottled water, 80
bowel cleansing, 168, 191
bowel movements, 90, 140
brachial plexus, 106
brahma-randra, 104
brain waves. *See* alpha brain waves; theta brain waves
breath: in *chi kung*, 99–100; in *kum nye*, 100–102
breathing: and digestion, 81; in healing meditation, 148, 149; in meditation, 144–45; and relaxation, 115; suppression of, 139; and Yantra Yoga, 113
Buddha in Tibetan Ayurveda, 25
Buddha of Aquamarine Light, 20
Buddha of Thailand, 122
Buddha Sakyamuni, 47
Buddha Vaidurya, 20
buddha-nature, 52
Buddhism, 15
Buddhist tantric practices, 110
butter, clarified. *See* ghee

caffeine, 32, 190, 191
calamus oil, 191
calamus root powder, 173
cancer, 99
carbohydrates, 57
carbon filters, 80
carbon monoxide, 80
case histories, 181–83, 190–93
castor oil, 172
cause and effect, 222
celibacy, 110, 111
cerebro-spinal fluid, 104, 105
Chakpori in Lhasa, 22–23
chakras, 59, 103, 106, 109, 183
Chalice Well of Glastonbury, 79
changes in lifestyle, 195, 212–13
changma, 183
channels, 129, 188
Charak Samhita, 167
charlatanism, 126
chemical dependency, 185–86
chemicals, 47, 76
chest pains, 163
chewing, 57–58, 81
chi, 81, 98, 103, 223–26, 239
chi kung, 99–100
chickpea flour, 93, 170
Chime Rinpoche, 11, 162
China: and acupuncture, 22; and *chi kung*, 99; cuisine of, 60; and herbal remedies, 82; Japanese takeover, 98; at medical conferences, 20; medicine of, 17, 23
Chinese astrology, 153
Chinese Astrology (Walters), 199
Chinese calendar, 200
Chinese Law of Five Transformations, 153
Chinese *tai chi*, 97
chlorine levels, 80
Choedhak, Dr. Tenzin, 85
Chogyam Trungpa Rinpoche, 11, 155, 161, 166
choices, 221
Choje Lama, 37
Chopel, Gedun. *Tibetan Arts of Love*, 130
chronic degenerative disease, 54
Chulen, 189–90
circulation, 169, 171
circulatory stimulation, 96, 105, 106
civilized interaction, 147, 151
clairvoyance, 183
clarified butter. *See* ghee

clarity, 215, 240
cleansing food, 78–79
cleansing practices, 21, 22, 186–87
Clear Light Publishers, 13
Clifford, Terry, *Tibetan Buddhist Medicine and Psychiatry*, 20, 94, 121, 128, 178, 233n.3
climates, 73, 196. *See also* seasons; weather
clinging, 221
clitoris, 129
clothing, 81
cocaine, 175
codependence, 155
Colbin, Annemarie, *Food and Healing*, 58, 76
colds, 54, 124, 135, 165, 174
colic, 76
colon, 95, 171, 239
colonics, 171
Communists, 98
compassion, 215, 239
competitive sports. *See* sports
Complete Guide to Nine-Star Ki, The (Sachs), 153, 200
computer terminals, 181
conception, 206
confidence in methods, 195
confidence in self, 195, 213
confusion, 26
congestion, 75, 93, 173
conscious incarnates, 217
consciousness, 217, 220, 222
consorts, 126
constipation, 137, 172, 191
constitutional types, 28–33, 218, 233–34n.3, 240 and exercise, 93, 94; as guide, 50–52; and *Len Nga*, 167–68, 187; and nutrition, 53–54; and spiritual practices, 141, 142
contemplation, 141
conventional health-care models, 19, 53
cosmetics, 124
cravings, 221
creative action, 142
crown point, 183
crying, 139
cultures, 40, 47, 73
cycles of time, 196

daily practices, 120–33
dairy products, 76, 77
Dalai Lama, 85, 97
days of the week, 204
delusions, 26
demineralized soils, 76
demonic possession, 178
denial, 26–27, 100
dependency, 221
dervish tradition, 103
desire, 163
detoxification, 12, 165–87, 198
Dharamsala, India, 85
Dharmaraksita, *Wheel of Sharp Weapons, The*, 132
diagnosis and treatment, 13
diarrhea, 90, 124, 136, 172
diet, 19, 53–92, 120; and exercise, 94; and season, 133, 134, 135, 136, 137
Diet for a New America (Robbins), 76
digestion: and breathing, 81; exercise, 93; and tongue coating, 125
digestive cleansing, 170–71
digestive fire, 58, 75, 89–92, 97, 135, 173, 240
digestive tract, 58
discriminations, 221
discursiveness of mind, 114, 115, 183–84
dissociation, 100
distillation, 80
distraction, 162
divinatory pulses, 37
dizziness, 103, 104, 163
DNA, 73
Doctrine of Interdependent Origination, 219
dog, 200–204
dog posture, 108
domesticated animals, 76
Donden, Dr. Yeshe, 12; and fragrances, 135; *Health Through Balance*, 37, 75, 92; on jogging, 94; and spiritual practices, 131; and virilification, 188
Dorje, Dr. Pema, 90
dosha, 27–33, 239
dough ring, 179
dragon, 200–204, 209
Dragon Rises, Red Bird Flies (Hammer), 23
draksha, 91
dreams, 122
drinking, 138
drops, 129
drugs, 32, 185, 222
dualistic split, 219, 220
dullness of mind, 162

Dummer, Dr. Tom, 12, 15; *Tibetan Medicine and Other Holistic Health-Care*, 90
dzub-nyin, 239

ear problems, 177
earth, 204, 224–25
earth observation, 197
eating, 138
ectomorphs, 29, 226
ego, 27, 119, 142, 161, 215
ego and suffering, 215–22
EIGHT White Earth, 159–60
ejaculation inhibition, 110, 111, 128, 129, 140
electric energy, 47
electro-encephalograms, 114
electromagnetic stimiuli, 47
elements of nature, 195–96, 199, 217, 224–25
elimination, 140, 169, 171
emesis. *See* vomiting
emotional states of *nyepas*, 225–26
emotions, 100, 221
endocrine balance, 58
endocrine functioning, 240
endocrines, 106
endomorphs, 30, 226
enemas, 21, 77, 171–72, 239
Energetics of Foods (Gagne), 76
energy flow, 59, 197
enlightenment, 28, 126, 131, 152, 188, 218, 220, 239–40
environment: connectedness to, 19, 51; forces of, 196; knowledge of, 121, 141; stress from, 47
enzymes, 74
epilepsy, 177
equanimity, meditation for, 144–47
Erlewhine, Michael, 199
ether, 224–25
ethics, 131–33
ethnicity, 40
eucalyptus, 169
excitability, 90
exercise, 19, 93–118, 120, 135, 136
existences, previous, 27
existential awareness, 148
Explanatory Tantra, 233
eyes, 163, 177, 179–83, 239

facial massage, 176
fall. *See* autumn
family lineage, 188
fasting, 63, 66
fatty foods, 90
favorable days, 204
fecal matter, 171
feelings, 221, 222
Feng Shi: The Chinese Art of Placement (Rossbach), 198
feng-shui, 197, 240
fertilizers, 76, 78
fevers, 172
fire, 204, 224–25, 240
"five actions," 140, 166–78, 239
"Five Rites," 102
"Five Tibetans," 102, 103
FIVE Yellow Earth, 157–58
fixated, 222
flexibility, 141, 142
flour cleansing technique, 93, 96, 135, 170, 185
flus, 54, 135, 165
flying, 183
food, 53–92; combinations of, 73–75; and exercise, 94; local sources of, 60; organic, 73, 77, 78; Oriental groceries, 60; quality of, 75–79; quantities of, 56; and seasons, 56, 133–34, 198; selection and preparation of, 58, 60; supplementations to 81–89
Food and Healing (Colbin), 76
Food Cleansing Formula One, 78–79
Food Cleansing Formula Two, 78–79
food industry, 77
footwear, 95
FOUR Green Space, 156–57
fragrances, 135, 136
freedom, 119
friendly days, 204
fruits, 74, 78
full-body isotonics, 98

Gagne, Stephen, *Energetics of Foods*, 76
gamma radiation, 76
Ganges, 79
garbanzo flour, 170
Garuda School of Tibet Tai Chi and Chuan Fa, 97, 100
gas, 137, 138, 139, 172, 191
gastrointestinal distress, 80
general behavior, 120–33

General Symptoms Test, 37–40
genetic engineering, 73
genetics, 208
genital region, 110–12
geomancy, 195, 196–98, 23, 240
ghee, 162, 171, 172, 173, 179, 239
ginger, 91, 162, 169, 175
glands, 101
global harmony, 77
goodness of man, 216
grains, 73–74, 78
Great Precious Accumulation Pill, The, 88
Greece, 17
green salads, 91
guided imagery in relaxation, 115, 118, 143
guilt, 147
Gulf War (Persian), 80
Gyud-Zhi, 12, 19–22, 120–21, 135, 233n.3, digestive fire, 91; exercise, 93; food, 75; oils, 124; sexual partners, 127–28; supression of natural urges, 138–40; water, 79–80

habitat, 197
habitual tendencies, 213, 222
half-lotus meditation pose, 146
Hammer, Dr. Leon, *Dragon Rises, Red Bird Flies*, 23
Hanaway, Pat 13
hand postures, 99
happiness, 119–20
hare, 200–204, 208
Hatha Yoga, 81
headaches, 136, 137, 172, 177, 178, 183
healing meditation, 147–53
Health Through Balance (Donden), 38, 75, 92
health-care practitioners, 13
heart disease, 99
Heart Sutra, 219
heat, 95, 96
hemorrhoids, 173, 190
herbal medicine, 17
herbs, 22; in second level of medicine, 21; selection of, 82; sources of, 60
hiccups, 138
high blood pressure, 178
Himalayas, 80
Hindu tantric practices, 110, 128
hing, 162
holistic health-care models, 19, 21
Holistic Medical Center (Lexington, Kentucky), 12
home setting, 197
homeopathy, 54, 92
homogenization, 77
homosexuals, 130
hormone levels, 76
horse, 200–204, 209
human potential, 141, 149, 166, 218
human predicament, 52
humors, 27–33, 213–16, 240
hybridization, 76
hydrotherapy, 168–70, 171, 185
hygiene, 124–25, 135
hyperactivity, 181
hypnosis, 143
hypothalamus, 57–58

I Ching trigram, 158
ice skating, 96
iced beverages, 90, 96, 136
ideal healer, 151
ignorace, 26–28, 30, 119, 164, 215–22, 233n.1, 239, 240
illusions, 120, 220
imagery, guided, 115, 118, 143
immune defense system, 103, 108, 137
impotence, 130
incest, 181–83
independence, 152
India, 17, 20, 60
Indian Ayurvedic tradition, 32, 166
indigestion, 53, 79, 90
individual responsibility, 54
individual spiritual orientation, 153–61
infant mortality rates, 54
infertility, 130
Inner Power: Secrets from Tibet and the Orient (Kilham), 102, 103, 111
insomnia, 191
internal organs, 105
intestinal tract, 169
invasiveness of therapies, 21–22, 53
inversion machines, 95, 135
isometric tensing, 107
isometrics and relaxation, 115, 118, 148
isotonics, full-body, 98

jamtsi, 171–72, 239
Japan, 98

Japanese astrology, 153
jealousy, 164
Jesus, 151
jogging, 94, 95, 135
Johari, Dr. Harish, *Ayurvedic Massage*, 168–69
joints, 169
Joshi, Dr. Sunil, 12, 173–74, 178
joy, 224
Joyous Lake (Tui), 158

Kalu Rinpoche, 128, 130
kapha, 28, 223–26
karma, 131, 240; and birth, 216–22
Karma Triyana dharmachakra, 15
kar-tse, 198, 239
Kelder, Peter, *Ancient Secrets of the Fountain of Youth*, 102, 109–10, 111
Khenpo Karthar Rinpoche, 11, 12, 15, 16, 162, 220–221
kichadi, 168, 191
kidneys, 110, 174–75, 177
Kilham, Christopher S., *Inner Power: Secrets from Tibet and the Orient*, 102, 103, 111
kinesiology, 85
klesa, 163, 219
kriya, 186
kum nye, 23, 100–102
Kunphen Tibetan Medical Hall and Clinic (Kathmandu), 86
Kushi, Michio, 11
Kuwait, 80
kyuk, 173–74, 239

Lad, Dr. Vasant, 12, 171
large intestine, 171
Lassalle, Rex, 11
leftovers, 75
leg lifts, 104–5
legumes, 73–74, 78
lemon water, 91
Len Nga therapy, 140, 166–78, 190–93, 198, 239, 240
lentil flour, 93, 96, 135
lethargic, 96
levitation, 183
Lhasa, 22–23
licorice tea, 173
life force, 81, 98, 103–4, 107, 174, 239, 240
lifestyles, 19, 22, 191; changes in, 195, 212–14; in first level of medicine, 21; management of, 17; and nutrition, 53; and psychotherapy, 192–93; in West, 47
lights flashing, 163
lime water, 91
"lion goes down the mountain," 99
lithium, 190
liver transplants, 76
loneliness of human existence, 148–49
longevity. *See* rejuvenation
lotus meditation pose, 145
LUNG, 28, 29, 47, 50, 191, 223–26, 239; and climate, 196; and colon or large intesinte, 171; and digestive fire, 91; and exercise, 95; food recommendations for, 60–63; and gas, 138; *Len Nga* process for, 186, 187; life force, 98, 174; massage for, 169; nasal therapy for, 174–75; and relaxation, 118; and seasons, 134, 137; and sesame oil, 93; and sex, 127, 128, 130; *Shiro dhara* for, 183; and sleep, 122; and tates, 55
LUNG-BEKAN, 69–72
LUNG-TrIPA combination, 69–72
lymph fluid, 169
lymphatic stimulation, 96, 135

macrobiotics, 11, 57, 58, 73
magnetic fields, 123
manic-depression, 190
Mantak Chia, 110
mantras, 16
marmas, 168–69, 223
martial arts, 11, 15, 97–100, 113, 168, 239
massage, 21–22, 100, 101, 113, 124, 239; facial, 176; in *Len Nga* therapy, 168–70, 171; and sleep, 123
masturbation, 130
"Matrix Software Tibetan Astrology Seminar" (Wangchuck), 153, 154, 199
meat eaters, 58–59
meats, 77, 90
medical tantras, 17, 20
medicinal plants, 21
Medicine Buddha, 12, 15, 16, 20, 120–21, 150, 151
meditation, 11, 17, 19, 22, 52, 103, 141–64; and alpha brain waves, 114; intensive practice of, 16, 189–90; problems in, 161–64; and relaxation, 115, 143; and

sex, 126; and *Shiro dhara*, 184
melons, 74
men and sex, 125, 126
menstruation, 83, 127, 128, 175
mental defilements, 163
mental distress, 171
mental obscurations, 163, 219
mental overstimulation, 183
mental problems, 93–94, 128, 193
mesomorphs, 30, 226
metabolic heat, 58, 75, 89–92, 97, 135, 137, 173, 240
metabolism, 224
mewas, 12, 153–61, 199, 201, 223
microorganisms, 80
migraines. *See* headaches
Milarepa Gampopa, 51–52
milk, 123
milk enemas, 77
mind, negative states of, 163–64
mind and body continuum, 208
mind dullness, 162
mind-body-spirit integration, 17, 25–26, 52, 99–100, 167
mindfulness, 11, 120, 121, 212
minerals, 53
mini-trampolines, 96, 135
miso soup, 91
mobility, 40
moisture levels, 133
monkey, 200–204, 210
monsoon season, 137
moon phases, 199
morality, 119, 120, 131–33
Morningstar, Amadea, *The Ayurvedic Cookbook*, 58, 75, 91
mortality, 148
motivation, 195, 213
mouse, 200–204, 207
movement, 223
moxabustion, 22
mucus, 75, 77, 93, 173
mudras, 99
music in relaxation, 115, 118

Na Jong, 174–77, 239
nadis, 183
Nagarjuna, 164
Naram, Dr. Pakanj, 12
nasal therapy, 174–77, 239
nasya, 191, 239
natural fibers, 81
natural food markets, 60
natural healing crisis, 92
natural therapies, 23
natural urges, repression of, 137–40
naturopathy, 17, 54, 92
nausea, 172
negative states of mind, 163
Nepal, 17, 189
nerve imbalances, 178
nerve plexuses, 101
nerves, 188
nervous system, 58, 105, 108, 239
Netra Basi, 179–83
neurolymphatic points, 168–69, 239
ngo drup, 183
nicotine, 190, 191
Nine House astrology of China, 11, 200
NINE Maroon Fire, 160
Nine-Star Ki system, 11–12, 200
Norbu, Namkhai, *Yantra Yoga*, 113
nose, 175
nuclear energy, 47
nutritional practices, 53–92. *See also* diet
nuts, 73–74
nyepas, 27–33, 223. *See also* constitutional types: classification of characteristics, 225–26; and exercise, 93–94; one dominant constitution, 29, 50; and tastes, 55–56; theory of, 223–26 two dominant constitutions, 29, 50, 69–72
Nyingma Institute, 101–2
nying-thig tsa-long, 100

obscurations, mental, 163, 219
occasional behavior, 137–40
oils, 124
Old Turquoise, 25, 89
Ole Nydahl, Lama, 11, 162, 216
ONE White Water, 154–55
openness, 142, 215
oral hygiene, 124–25
oral sex, 130
Oral tradition Tantra, 233
orgasmic fluid, 110
out-of-body experiences, 114
overeating, 90
overheating, 136
overplanted soils, 76

overweight, 96
ox, 200–204, 207
oxygen levels, 80
ozone depletion, 80

pains, shooting, 163
palpitation, 163
Pancha Karma therapy, 17, 140, 166–78, 187, 239
Parcells, Dr. Hazel, 78
parents, 217, 220
penis, 129
perceptions, 26
Persia, 17, 20
Persian Gulf War, 80
Personality Profile Test, 33, 41–46
perspiration, 90, 95–96, 97, 135, 136
pesticides, 76, 78
petro-chemicals, 80, 124
petroleum-based waxes, 76
pharmacology, 21, 82
phlegm, 224, 239
pho thut, 58, 75, 89–92, 97, 135, 173, 240
physical labor, 93, 94
pig, 200–204, 212
pitta, 28, 223–26
placement. *See* geomancy
plants, medicinal, 21
Pon Tsang Zana, 89
Power Eating Program, The (Stanchich), 57–58
pragmatic approach, 23
prakruti, 218, 240
Prakruti (Svaboda), 49
prana, 98, 174, 240
precious ones, 217
Precious Pills, Tibetan, 85–89
pregnancy, 173–74, 175
pregnant women, 127, 128
prepared frozen meals, 76
preventative health care, 11, 13, 19–23, 55, 187, 213
previous existences, 27, 217
pride, 164, 219
privacy, 21
processed foods, 75, 90
"Profound Inner Meaning, The," 188
proteins, animal, 74; metabolism of, 57; vegetable, 74; whole, 73
psychic energies, 103
psychic network, 188
psychological faculties of *nyepas*, 225
"psycho-spiritual" massage, 183
psychotherapy, 181–83, 190–93
psychotic episodes, 171
pulse diagnosis, 85
pulse taking, 37–38, 92
pungent, 55
purgation, 21, 136, 172–73
purification, body, 137, 140, 186
purification systems, in-home, 80
Purified Moon Crystal, 86–88
purple cabbage, 75
quality of food, 75–79
quantites of food, 56

race, 40
racket sports, 96
radical medical interventions, 40
radioactive stimuli, 47
rang-zhin. See constitutional types
Rapgay, Dr. Lobsang, 12, 17–18; *Chulen* prescriptions, 190; days of the week, 201–2; healing meditation, 147–53; and *Len Nga* therapy, 167; medication problems, 162; *pho thut*, 91; relaxation exercise, 115–18; *Shiro dhara*, 183; Tibetan Personality Profile, 41: urine testing, 83–85; and Yantra Yoga, 112–13
rasayanas, 189
reality, 15, 26, 31, 215, 221
rebounders, 96
rectum, 172
red blood cells, 169
regional cuisines, 73
reincarnation, 217–22
rejuvenation, 12, 13, 19, 22, 23, 165–66, 188–93, 239; exercises, 102–12
Relative World, Ultimate Mind (Tai Situ Rinpoche), 51, 197, 199, 217
relaxation, 19, 81, 167; and *kum nye*, 100–102; and meditation, 115, 143
relaxation therapy, 113–18
religions, 142
religious zealots, 143
REM sleep, 114, 121
renutrification, 77, 165
reoxygenation, 99–100, 169
repa, 189
repression of natural urges, 137–40
responsibility, individual, 54, 141

retreats, 184, 189, 214
reverse osmosis, 80
Rigpe Yeshe, 20, 233n.3
Rinchen Mangjor Chenmo (The Great Precious Accumulation Pill), 88
Rinchen Ratna Samphel (Recious Wish Fulfilling Jewel), 88
Rinchen Repa, 189–90
Rinchen Tso-Tru Dhashel (Precious Purified Moon Crystal), 86–88
Rinchen Yu Nying, 25, 89
Rinpoches, 217
rituals in fourth level of medicine, 22
Robbins, John, *Diet for a New America*, 76
roma, 183
Root Tantra, 233
Rossbach, Sarah, *Feng Shui: The Chinese Art of Placement*, 198
running. *See* jogging
rural, 54

sache, 197, 240
Sachs, Melanie, 12–13, 15; *Ayurvedic Beauty Care*, 101, 124, 136; nasal therapy procedure, 175–77
Sachs, Robert, *Complete Guide to Nine-Star Ki, The*, 153, 200
sacral pump mechanism, 105
saffron, 77
saints, 29, 31, 51
saliva, 139
salivary amylase, 57
salty, 55
sanitation, 54, 80
Sanskrit, 28
scalp sensitivity, 183
seasons, *See also* climates; weather: and behavior, 133–37, 198; and exercise, 94, 96–97; and food, 56, 73; and sex, 129
seeds, 73–74
self-actualization, 166, 217
self-esteem, 120, 132, 193
self-evaluation, 25–52
self-fulfillment, 25
self-limitations, 218, 219
self-massage, 100, 101, 113
self-reflection, 141
semen, 110, 128
seminars, 16, 214
senior citizens, 54
senna tea, 172
sense fields, 218, 220
sesame oil: for enemas, 171; and exercise, 93, 95, 96; in massage, 168, 175; in *Shiro dhara*, 183, 240; and sleep, 123
setting, 195, 196–98
SEVEN Red Air, 158–59
sex and men, 125, 126
sex and women, 125, 126, 127, 128
sexual acts, 130
sexual aggrandizement, 126
sexual behavior, 120, 121
sexual fluid retention, 128, 129
sexual force, 129, 189
sexual foreplay, 130
sexual intercourse, 110, 111, 125–30
sexual intercourse postures, 130
sexual organs, 110–12
sexual partners, 127–28, 189
shamanic system of medicine, 17
Shambhala Training, 11, 161
Shaolin Temple, 97–98
sheep, 200–204, 210
shel, 172
shiatsu, 11, 181, 190, 239
shipment of foods, 73
Shiro dhara, 183–86, 191, 240
shooting pains, 163
shoulder problems, 107
siddhis, 183
Sierra States University School of Nutrition, 78
siestas, 123
Silk Road, 20
sinus cavities, 173, 174, 175, 177, 190
SIX White Air, 158
skillful activity, 215
skillful behavior, 119–40
skillful means, 125–26
skin disorders, 174, 178
skull bones, 57
sleep, 121–23, 139, 185
small intestine, 171, 240
snake, 200–204, 209
sneezing, 139
soaps, 124
soccer, 96
social environment, 213
social support, 212–14
soils, 76

sok lung, 174, 240
solar plexus, 107
solid food, 56
solidity, 223
sound in relaxation, 115
sour, 55
spaced out, 162–63, 222
species interdependence, 77
Specific Symptoms Observed Over Time Test, 47–49
spices, 60, 75
spinal flexibility, 96
spine stretching, 104–5, 108
spinning, 103–4
spirit-body-mind integration, 17, 25–26, 52, 99–100, 167
spiritual medicine, fourth level, 22, 27
spiritual practices, 17, 131–33, 141–65
spiritual work, 19, 51–52
spitting, 139
sports, 93, 94, 95, 96
spring, 135–36
Stanchich, Lino, *The Power Eating Program*, 57–58
starches, 57
starry formations, 163
Stature and Physical Characteristics Test, 35–36
steam boxes, 169
steam rooms, 169
"stepping over rocks," 99
stillness, 100
Stoll, Dr. Walt, 12
stomach, 56, 171, 173
stress, 95, 97, 170
stress-related illnesses, 99, 114
stretching, 95; of spine, 104–5
Strongstan Gampo, King, 20
Subsequent Tantra, 233
suffering and ego, 215–22
Sufism, 103
suicide, 190
summer, 136
sunlight, 133
supermarkets, 60
supportive network, 195, 212–14
surgery, 21, 22
Surkhar Nyam-Nyi Dorjee, 86
survival skills, 26
Svaboda, Dr. Robert, Prakruti, 49
sweat lodges, 169
sweating. *See* perspiration
sweet, 55
swimming, 96, 121
symptoms in constitutional determination, 39–40

table pose, 107
tabula rasa, 222
tai chi, 11, 23, 95, 97–99
Tai Situ Rinpoche, *Relative World, Ultimate Mind*, 51, 197, 199, 217
Tanatuk, 20
tantras, 17, 20
tantric sexual union, 126
Tao of Love, 155
Taoist practices, 110, 128, 166
Tarthang Tulku Rinpoche, 100–102
tastes, 55–56, 57
tastes and seasons, 134, 135, 137
temporal lobes of skull, 57
tension headaches. *See* headaches
tests: to determine constitutional types, 31–49; scoring of, 33–34
thankas, 126
theta brain waves, 184
third eye, 183, 184, 240
Third Karmapa's treatise, 188
thirst, 90
THREE Blue Space, 155–56
three *nyepas* in balance constitutions, 29, 50–51
Three Poisons, 26–28, 50–52, 120, 121, 141, 142, 215–17, 233, 239, 240
throat, 175
throat mucus, 139
thryoid, 106
thymus, 106
Tibet, cuisine of, 58, 60
Tibet, historical perspective, 17, 23, 58, 60
Tibet, holistic medical capital of Asia, 20
Tibetan Arts of Love, (Chopel), 130
Tibetan astrology, 153–61
Tibetan Ayurveda, 25–26, 47, 166
Tibetan Ayurvedic health practitioners, 32
Tibetan Buddhist Medicine and Psychiatry (Clifford), 20, 94, 121, 128, 178, 233
Tibetan calendar, 200
Tibetan Medical and Astro Institute, 86
Tibetan Medical Center, 85
Tibetan medicine, 13, 15, 17–18, 19–23, 53, 233n.3

Tibetan medicine and Other Holistic Health–care (Dummer), 12, 90
Tibetan Personality Profile Test, 33, 41–46
Tibetan Precious Pills, 85–89
Tibetan Rejuvenation Exercises, 102–12
tiger, 200–204, 208
timing, 195, 196, 198–204
tiredness, 75, 90
tongue coating, 124–25
toxic waste, 47
toxins, 169, 170
transformations. *See* elements of nature
transplants, 222
travel, 47
trifala, 168
trikatu, 91
TrIPA, 28, 30, 50, 223–26, 240; and blood-letting, 178; and climate, 196; and digestive fire, 91; and exercise, 95–96; food recommendations for, 63–66; *Len Nga* process for, 187; massage for, 169; and relaxation, 118; and seasons, 136; small intestine, 171; and tastes, 55
TrIPA-BEKAN, 69–72
Trogawa Rinpoche, 12
trul-khor, 113
tsampa, 58
tsothel, 85
tuberculosis, 174
tulkus, 217
Twelve Nidamas, 219–22, 240
twelve-year cycle of archetypal energy patterns, 199
TWO Black Earth, 155
Type A personalities, 30

undergarments, 81
urination, 140, 177
urine testing, 83–85, 92
urine testing in constitutional determination, 39

Vajrayana, 15
vascular system, 178
vata, 28, 223–26, 239
vegetables, 78
vestibular system, 103
vibrancy, 223
victims, 119
violence, 125
virilification practices, 130, 166, 188
vision quests, 184
vistas, 96
visual memories, 182
visualization, 16, 143–44, 147
vitamins, 53, 82
vomina, 239
vomiting, 21, 123, 135, 139, 163, 173–74, 239
vulnerability, 148

walking, 95, 135
Walters, Derek, *Chinese Astrology*,199
Wangchuck, Sangye, "Matrix Software Tibetan Astrology Seminar," 153, 154, 199
warm water, 53, 79, 91
water, 79–80, 96, 224–25
weak women, 127, 128
weather, 95. *See also* seasons; climates
Western medical community, 19
Westerners, 40, 47
Wheel of Sharp Weapons, The (Dharmaraksita), 132
Willful intent, 211
wind, 129, 188, 224, 239
wines, 91
winter, 134
wisdom, 125–26, 215
Wisdom channel, 149
Wish Fulfilling Jewel, 88
women and sex, 125, 126, 127, 128
Wood, Rebecca, 58

yab-yum, 126
yang, 98, 99, 223–26, 240
Yantra Yoga, 17, 112
Yantra Yoga (Norbu), 113
yawning, 138
year of birth, 153
Yellow Emperor's Classic of Internal Medicine, 81
Yile Kye, 20, 233n.3
yin and *yang*, 153, 223–26
yoga, 95, 100, 102, 105, 107
yogic traditions, 110, 113, 122
yogis, 189
Yutok Yoten Gonpo, 17

zealots, religious, 143

BOOKS OF RELATED INTEREST FROM NAB

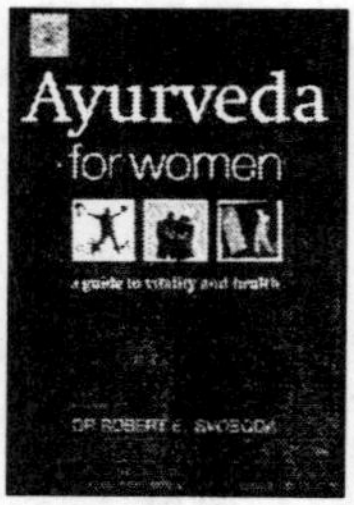

AYURVEDA FOR WOMEN: A Guide to Vitality and Health—*Dr. Robert E. Svoboda*

Focusing on the modern woman's need to heal and empower her body, mind and spirit in a fast-moving world, this fascinating new book explains the principles of a system of complementary medicine that is rapidly gaining in popularity. Besides, it offers practical advice to women of all ages on applying those principles in everyday life and also provides essential reading for all women interested in maintaining good health—through simple, natural methods and complementary therapies.

ISBN: 978-81-7822-105-2

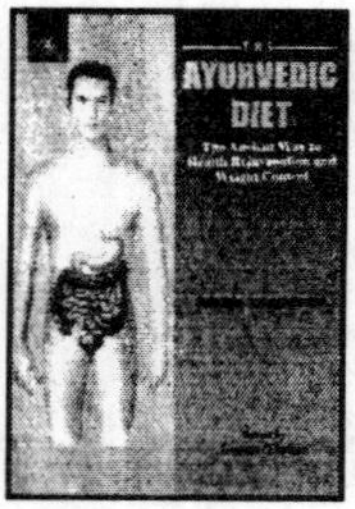

THE AYURVEDIC DIET: The Ancient Way to Health Rejuvenation and Weight Control —*Dennis Thompson*

The Ayurvedic Diet combines the ancient wisdom of Ayurveda for health and healing with modern scientific approach to body physiology. This book offers practical solutions for everything from chronic health problems and weight control to the proper exercise and life style management. It is essential reading for all who want to lose weight, stay young and be healthy.

ISBN: 978-81-7822-014-7

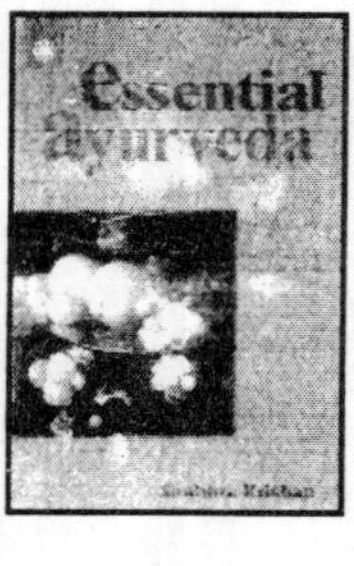

ESSENTIAL AYURVEDA: What it is & What it Can do for You —*Shubhra Krishan*

Perhaps the oldest healing tradition in the world, Ayurveda is based on maintaining harmony of the mind, body, and spirit for optimal wellness, and can easily be incorporated into today's life-styles. Peppered with healthful recipes and tips, this book has been written with your questions and concerns in mind. It demystifies Ayurveda, showing it as a prevention-oriented, do-it-yourself system of healing.

ISBN: 978-81-7822-216-5